"Using a short question-and blends the technical with the humorous for a fun and engaging read . . . a very informative and interesting book for men and women. Recommended for public libraries."
—Library Journal

". . . smart, funny and informative. It should be required reading for any man who cares about women.
—Marilu Henner
actress and New York Times best-selling
author, *Marilu Henner's Total Makeover*

"We finally have a guide for men to understand female complexities. . . . I recommend it highly."
—Harold H. Bloomfield, M.D.
Psychiatrist and best-selling author,
Making Peace with Your Past

"This isn't a book just for men. I've rarely seen a resource with this much information about gynecology. It should be in every library—personal and public—in the country."
—Pat Heim, Ph.D.
President, the Heim Group
Lecturer and author, *Smashing the Glass Ceiling*

". . . reference source that is a superb combination of succinct technical information blended with a witty, down-to-earth writing style that you will enjoy reading."
—Robert Israel, M.D.
Professor and chief, Gynecology,
Department of Obstetrics and Gynecology,
USC School of Medicine

"I think women can probably learn a lot of things from this book, too. I know I could"

—Jodi Applegate
Later Today, NBC-TV

"Digestible, to the point, full of truth and very funny. *Your Guy's Guide to Gynecology* is a wonderful way to approach those topics and situations that make us all squirm."

—Kate Jennison
National Post (Canada)

". . . an easy-to-read, practical, balanced, and informative guide to the body you love and the woman you cherish."

—Warren Farrell, Ph.D.
Author, *Why Men Are The Way They Are*
and *Women Can't Hear What Men Don't Say*

"With this humorous, easy-to-read and authoritative book, Drs. Bekkar and Wahn provide the essentials for understanding women's health issues."

—John Gray
Author, *Men Are from Mars, Women Are from Venus*

"An important book whose time has come."

—Dr. Drew Pinsky
Co-host of "Loveline" MTV and Radio,
author, *The Dr. Drew and Adam Book*

"A witty approach to women's health . . . easily readable and keeps one's attention . . . very thorough and (handles) some very touchy subjects in a very gentle and sensitive way."

—Katherine Sheehan, M.D.
Medical Director, Planned Parenthood
of San Diego and Riverside Counties

"Readers–men, women, and health care professionals of all kinds–should find this book an overdue resource that helps to demystify gynecology, a subject that has been taboo for too long."

—*The Permanente Journal*

"It's very well written and a useful resource."

—**Kathryn DeMott**
Editor, *Ob. Gyn. News*

"This book is fun, enjoyable, and easy to read. Bekkar and Wahn have made a complex subject understandable. I only wish I had this information earlier. Excellent. Women, buy this book. Men, read it."

—**Dick Roth**
Author, *"No, It's Not Hot In Here": A Husband's Guide to Understanding Menopause*

"Not just for guys—this is a must-read for couples. A great opportunity to have open discussion between the sexes. This should help demystify the gynecologist's office for the partners of our patients.

—**Raquel D. Arias, M.D.**
Associate Dean for Women &
Associate Professor of Obstetrics and Gynecology
U.S.C. School of Medicine

"Drs. Bekkar and Wahn demystify what gynecology is all about and help the reader obtain a deeper understanding of what makes a woman tick."

—**Howard E. Richmond, M.D.**
Psychiatrist and Psychotherapist
Clinical Faculty
University of California San Diego College of Medicine

"A wonderful recipe for intimacy and understanding in relationships plus a 'must have' health resource for your personal library."

—Diana von Welanetz Wentworth
Co-author, *Chicken Soup for the Soul Cookbook*
Founder, The Inside Edge

"Understanding is a critical part of caring. *Your Guy's Guide to Gynecology* provides a concise and humorous response to Professor Higgins's question: Why can't a woman be more like a man? For many men it may be an aid to improved relationships; for others it may be the key to their survival. Don't let this opportunity for enlightenment pass you by!"

—Peter McGough, M.D.
Past-president, Washington State Medical Association
Washington Physicians for Social Responsibility

"Every guy should read this book and save it forever as a reference. Every woman will want to buy it for her guy (and I bet read it herself)."

—Lila Nachtigall, M.D.
Professor, Obstetrics & Gynecology,
NYU School of Medicine, Director of Women's Wellness at NYU
President, The North American Menopause Society
Author, *Estrogen: The Facts Can Change Your Life*

"Dr. Bruce is loving, wise, insightful, brilliant, and as funny as Dave Barry. You'll love this book!"

—Mark Victor Hansen
Co-creator, the #1 New York Times best-selling series
Chicken Soup For The Soul™

Your Guy's Guide to Gynecology

Your Guy's Guide to Gynecology

Everything You Wish He Knew About Your Body If He Wasn't Afraid to Ask

BRUCE BEKKAR, MD
UDO WAHN, MD

Ant Hill Press
Sandwich, Massachusetts

For permissions and reprint information, contact:
North Star Publications/Ant Hill Press
P.O. Box 227 • East Sandwich, MA 02537-0227
Tel (508) 420-6188 • Fax (508) 420-6570
email norbook@aol.com • www.anthillpress.com

Printed in U.S.A.

First Printing — January 2001; ISBN 0-9655067-7-0

Jacket design: Nichole Smith • Jacket photos: © Photodisc
Interior illustrations: Steve Troop

Disclaimer
This book is a reference work and is intended for the general reading public and not as a substitute for qualified medical care. Care has been taken to confirm the accuracy of the information presented and to describe generally accepted practices. However, the authors, editors, and publisher are not responsible for errors or omissions or for any consequences from application of the information in this book and make no warranty, expressed or implied, with respect to the contents of the publication.

Publisher's Cataloging-in-Publication
Bekkar, Bruce.
        Your guy's guide to gynecology / Bruce Bekkar, Udo
        Wahn. — 1st ed.
                p.   cm.
        Includes bibliographic references and index.
        ISBN:
        1. Gynecology—Popular works. 2. Women—Health and
        hygiene. I. Wahn, Udo. II. Title.
RG121.B45   2000   618.1
                                              QBI00-94

CONTENTS

FOREWORD

In today's world, men must understand and be sensitive to the needs of women. How is this accomplished? First, it must be important to you and, second, you must read this book.

Doctors Bekkar and Wahn have made a major contribution to lessening the "War of the Roses." They have taken gynecology, the medical speciality that deals with disease and care of the female reproductive system, and made it practical and understandable. If Adam had read this book *before* he entered the Garden, this effort would be superfluous now, but he didn't, and it isn't. . . .

Obstetrics, the medical specialty that deals with birth and its antecedents and sequelae, gets all the publicity. There are a plethora of books, tapes, and CDs for expectant mothers, fathers, siblings, and grandparents on all pregnancy-related topics. The involved male has nine months to do the right thing.

Finally, men who want to do the right thing have a complete reference on gynecology written just for them. This book is a superb source of succinct technical information blended with a witty, down-to-earth writing style that you will enjoy reading.

To be a successful, enlightened gynecologist, or a successful, communicating male, you have to be part psychiatrist. Cyclicity, or the lack thereof, between the female reproductive system is the major physiologic link that dictates all "basic female stuff." If you understand this concept then you are well on your way, and this book will help you complete your journey. The nice thing about owning it, and it should be a reference source in *your* library, not borrowed sporadically from the local library, is that it can grow old as the women you know gracefully age. Right now, "Bumps, Drips, and Owies" may be your primary concern, but years from now your frayed copy will still be there when you need to know how to repel the "Attack of the Killer Hormones."

Although the book is for the "hulking beasts," the authors have cleverly entitled it *Your Guy's Guide to Gynecology*. Drs. Bekkar and Wahn know *who* is going to buy this guide and give it to those who think "a vulva is a Swedish sports sedan." Without a doubt, they have filled a void in many bookshelves and many lives. If you are reading this foreword, start spreading the news.

—Robert Israel, MD, Professor, Chief, Gynecology
Department of Obstetrics and Gynecology
University of Southern California School of Medicine

PREFACE

A BOOK ABOUT GYNECOLOGY *FOR GUYS??*

To the best of our knowledge, such a book has never been written before. Why did two busy gynecologists bother to take the time to write this book? Were we bored, were the tennis courts all booked, did we just need an alternate income source because of looming health care reform? Yes, but there's a better reason:

In the arena of traditional male/female relationships, nothing is more important than *communication* and *understanding*.

Men have been slowly learning to communicate with women, aided by some recent books, seminars, and the gentle urgings of their partners. Gradually, we hulking beasts are learning to open up and talk about our feelings, to develop our so-called feminine sides. Despite these heroic efforts, men don't always *understand* women.

One area in which this is particularly true is women's reproductive health, areas such as contraception, Pap smears, and fertility. As gynecologists, we have learned that most guys have only a superficial understanding of their partner's reproductive anatomy. This is unfortunate, because reproductive health issues are very important in relationships. At the least, when your wife or girlfriend visits the gynecologist, she must endure a highly personal and often uncomfortable examination. Our patients often tell us that they would appreciate more understanding from you, their partners.

But let's face it, guys. Most of you wouldn't know a Pap smear from a reindeer. You probably think that a vulva is a Swedish sports sedan. You know your girlfriend's got PMS, but you'd rather join the Witness Relocation Program than learn anything about it. The long and short of it is, when she comes home from the gynecologist, trying to discuss the exam with you is like trying to get the Pope to do a condom commercial.

What you might not have realized is that your partner's reproductive health affects *you* directly. Her choice of birth control will be a major factor in your sex life together. If she has a disease called endometriosis, she may be *unable* to make love because of pain. Some types of pelvic infections may make her sterile. Gynecologic surgery may cause temporary and/or long-term changes in your relationship. Certainly, if you've ever been involved with a woman with PMS, you know it affects both of you. We wrote this book to help you better understand your partner's reproductive physiology and be more supportive if she develops female health problems.

The first chapter of *Your Guy's Guide to Gynecology* is called "Basic Female Stuff." The chapter begins with a short course on female reproductive anatomy. Next we explain how all those structures work together in the menstrual cycle. You'll learn something about menstrual periods, the potent female hormone estrogen, and fertility.

The next chapter, "Let's Talk about Sex, Baby," covers two often-overlooked areas for guys: contraception and female sexual response. In these pages, you'll learn about the birth control method you are using. You can also check out others you may be curious about. If you *really* want to impress your mate, we suggest you read the section on female sexual response. Here you'll find practical hints for having a happy long-term physical relationship.

In "Vaginitis" and "Bumps, Drips, and Owies," we investigate vaginal infections and sexually transmitted diseases. In these two chapters, you'll find useful information on the diagnosis and treatment of common vaginal infections such as yeast and trichomoniasis, as well as more serious infections such as chlamydia, gonorrhea, venereal warts, herpes, and syphilis. Most importantly, you'll find out how to keep yourself and your partner from getting these infections.

The fifth chapter of *Your Guy's Guide to Gynecology* covers the most dangerous infection of all: HIV/AIDS. What you learn here may save your life.

In Chapter 6, "Attack of the Killer Hormones," we bring you up-to-date on PMS and the menopause. And since your behavior is crucial to your relationship if either of these problems exists, we provide lots of suggestions: what to do if your partner has PMS, what you can do for a woman going through the menopause, and our own "Top Ten List of Things We Don't Recommend You Say to a Woman with PMS."

Chapter 7, "Complicated Female Stuff Made Simple," explains the mysteries of bladder infections, breast lumps, abnormal Pap smears, endometriosis, and fibroid tumors of the uterus. In a long-term relationship, most guys will encounter one or more of these problems with their mates. We teach you what you'll need to know and how to respond to her in ways she'll really appreciate.

In "Under the Knife: Gynecologic Surgery," we review state-of-the-art gynecologic surgery: the D & C, surgery for ovarian cysts and ectopic pregnancy, and hysterectomy. Risks, benefits, and alternative treatments are covered. For those who are interested, we'll even describe how each operation is performed. Perhaps most important, tips on how you can help your partner through her operation and recovery are found at the end of the chapter.

Chapter 9 deals with pregnancy. These days, many couples ask us how to prepare for having a child. We hear questions like "What should I be eating?" "How about exercise?" and "Should I stop my medications?" Once we can get the *guys* to quit talking, we ask their wives what *they* want to know. The answers are all found in Chapter 9, "So, You Want to Have a Baby."

Finally we disclose what happens when a woman goes to the gynecologist for a pelvic exam. At last you'll understand why most women truly dislike visiting their gynecologist.

You'll find all the information in *Your Guy's Guide to Gynecology* useful and interesting. Also, we have labored to bring it to you in a way that won't make you feel like you're reading a textbook:

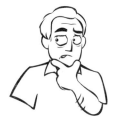

- At the start of each chapter, you can test your knowledge of the topics to be covered by taking a brief "Guy-Q Test."

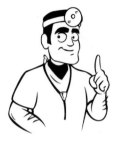

- Within the chapters, you'll often see a friendly young doctor in the margins. These sections, called "Doc Talk," highlight important points to remember. We also might relate a story about a particularly unusual patient we've cared for.

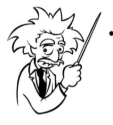

- Whenever you see the professor, we're about to present some technical information. We might describe a procedure we perform, or refer to clinical studies to clarify a point. You can read these sections if you're interested, or just skip over them if you're not.

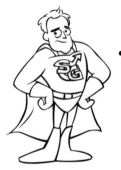

- Our favorite character is Supportive Guy. He provides suggestions for how to help your partner through some of the health problems we describe. Pay particular attention to what he says—you'll both be glad you did.

At the end of each chapter, a short Post Test checks to see if you learned the basic points we covered.

A word about our credentials: We are Board-Certified OB-GYN physicians with training in both public and private hospitals. We have more than 25 years of clinical experience between us, and maintain busy practices with a large and progressive HMO in Southern California.

We feel both honored and challenged by our work as physicians at the dawn of this new century. *Your Guy's Guide to Gynecology* is our attempt to make men better informed, and help bring couples closer together during the times of stress that illness often produces. We applaud your willingness to learn about this important topic, and we hope that our book is helpful.

Bruce Bekkar, MD
Udo Wahn, MD

P.S. If you *aren't* in a relationship now and can't find a reason to read this book, we suggest you go to a nearby Starbuck's, order a Mocha-whatever, and just start reading it anyway. You won't be alone for long . . .

BASIC FEMALE STUFF

CONFUSED (from Webster's): to be mixed up, disordered, thrown together indiscriminately, jumbled.

Judging by the comments we get from our patients, most guys are a little confused about female anatomy. The uterus, fallopian tubes, and ovaries are just mysterious "parts" to them. This certainly makes it unlikely these guys would understand subjects of practical importance, like the menstrual cycle, fertility, and female sexual response.

Your Guy's Guide to Gynecology seeks to narrow this information gap. Our first task in this introductory chapter is to cover female reproductive anatomy. So you won't feel bad if you're a bit clueless in this area, we start off with excerpts from an all-male focus group. We took a group of typical guys and asked them to draw what they believed to be "women's parts." After you see what they came up with, you'll feel better if you're not exactly an expert in this area.

After discussing the focus group, we get down to business with useful information on female reproductive anatomy. You will find the drawings and descriptions handy as you read the rest of *Your Guy's Guide to Gynecology*.

What follows this brief anatomy lesson is some physiology: How do all these "parts" work together? How do the ovaries, uterus, and brain communicate to ready a woman's body for pregnancy each month? In the section on the **menstrual cycle**, you'll find out what a period actually is, a little about the potent female hormone estrogen, and how to predict when your partner will be fertile each month.

Although it's not necessary to become an expert, some understanding of these topics shows care and concern for the woman you love. This knowledge will also be helpful when you're being physically intimate—or if she develops a physical problem.

We hope that you enjoy "Basic Female Stuff." Reading this chapter will prepare you for much of what follows in *Your Guy's Guide to Gynecology.*

GUY-Q TEST

1. The uterus is:
   a. the organ where menstrual bleeding originates from each month.
   b. the place where a baby grows until it is born.
   c. made mostly of muscle tissue.
   d. all of the above.

2. True statements about the cervix include:
   a. It is the lower or vaginal end of the uterus.
   b. The cervix can be seen at the top of the vagina.
   c. Pap smears are taken from this site to check for cancer.
   d. all of the above.

3. A woman's ovaries:
   a. produce powerful hormones: estrogen and progesterone.
   b. are the place where fertilized eggs grow.
   c. are located within the fallopian tubes.

4. Which of the following is *not* a part of female reproductive anatomy?
   a. Vulva
   b. Vas deferens
   c. Labia minora
   d. Fallopian tubes

5. The normal menstrual cycle is typified by:
   a. fluctuations in thyroid hormone levels.
   b. a regular interval of 21 to 35 days from one cycle to the next.
   c. bleeding at unpredictable intervals.

6. Estrogen has the following effects in women:
   a. It stimulates growth of breast tissue during puberty.
   b. It causes buildup of the inner lining of the uterus (the endometrium) each month in preparation for pregnancy.
   c. It can cause overgrowth of the clitoris.
   d. a and b only.

7. Menstrual periods are the result of:
   a. millions of eggs released by the ovaries.
   b. the brain stimulating the uterus to prevent pregnancy.
   c. the shedding of unused lining of the uterus when conception fails to occur.

8. During a pelvic exam, a gynecologist will usually examine the following:
   a. The area outside the vagina
   b. The vagina and the cervix
   c. The uterus, ovaries, and tubes
   d. All of the above

9. A speculum is:
   a. used to obtain Pap smears.
   b. a medical instrument that allows examination of the vagina.
   c. used to check hearing and eyesight.
   d. a and b only.

10. A visit to the gynecologist may include:
    a. a breast examination.
    b. a pelvic examination.
    c. a thorough review of past medical and surgical history.
    d. all of the above.

Key: 1. d   2. d   3. a   4. b   5. b   6. d   7. c   8. d   9. d   10. d

FOCUS GROUP

In an effort to decide whether our patients were correct in their assertion that men knew very little about female anatomy, we convened a focus group. We selected a small group of men from 25 to 55 years old who met our criteria: they could be bribed with a free dinner into exposing what they knew, or didn't know, about women's anatomy.

We believed that if men didn't have this level of basic knowledge, they couldn't possibly understand women's reproductive physiology. They wouldn't be equipped to discuss birth control or fertility planning; problems like PMS and abnormal Pap smears would be mysterious as well.

After a brief introduction, we decided to find out. With fingers crossed, we gave each participant a blank sheet of paper and a pencil. Our instructions to them were to draw and label, as accurately as they could, the female reproductive system.

After twenty minutes, we collected the papers. The drawings were scored according to how *inaccurate* they were; sadly, there was a lot of competition for first place. Here are some of the actual illustrations:

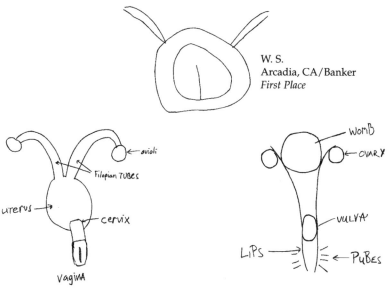

W. S.
Arcadia, CA/Banker
First Place

M. P.
New York/Computer Consultant
Second Place

C. W. P.
Middletown, PA/Administrator
Third Place

Now, it's your turn! Draw the female reproductive system in the space below. Be as complete and accurate as you can. Once you're finished, check your work against Figure 1.2, in the next section. Remember, this knowledge is just the *first* step in understanding your partner's reproductive physiology.

FEMALE ANATOMY

Women's reproductive anatomy is clearly quite different from men's. The good news is that it's not difficult to master the basics. After these next few pages, topics like estrogen, menstrual cycles, and even uterine fibroids won't be all that mysterious.

We'll begin with the external reproductive structures:

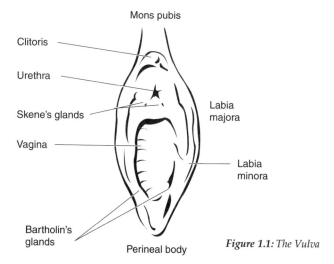

Mons pubis

Clitoris

Urethra

Skene's glands

Vagina

Labia majora

Labia minora

Bartholin's glands

Perineal body

Figure 1.1: The Vulva

Vulva

The vulva is the area outside of the vagina. Figure 1.1 highlights the following features of the vulva:

- **Mons pubis** The area just above the vagina, the *mons*, or mound, of slightly raised tissue where the pubic hair is the thickest.

- **Labia minora** The thin set of "lips" that surrounds the opening of the vagina.

- **Labia majora** Just lateral to the labia minora, these broad labia are slightly raised, like the mons pubis. Beneath them lie connective tissue and a small cushion of fat.

- **Perineal body** The delicate skin just below the vaginal entrance and above the rectum. This is where episiotomies are made to enlarge the vaginal opening at the time of birth.

- **Bartholin's and Skene's glands**   These glands lie beneath the skin and secrete lubricating fluid into the vagina; when blocked, they can become extremely painful and swollen.

- **Urethra**   The urethra is the opening for the urinary bladder. Its short length (much shorter than in men) and close proximity to the vagina explain why bladder infections so often occur after sex: vaginal bacteria can be pushed up into the bladder during intercourse.

- **Clitoris**   The clitoris lies at the top of the vagina, beneath the fusion (joining) of the labia minora. A similar structure in men is the glans penis—the head of the penis. *Both* are exquisitely sensitive to touch and must be treated gently. Appropriate stimulation of the clitoris is often necessary for a woman to achieve orgasm.

Vagina

The vagina is a tubular structure leading to the uterus and the upper genital tract. It is lined by a specialized, highly sensitive skin, and is capable of stretching and dilating to allow for childbirth. Remarkably, it returns to much of its prior size and shape afterward.

The vagina plays host to many types of microorganisms. These microorganisms usually live in harmony, but occasionally the balance is upset, one species overgrows, and painful symptoms of vaginitis soon follow.

Uterus

The uterus, also known as the womb, is a sacklike muscular structure about the size and shape of a pear. It is located just above the vagina in the lower part of the abdominal cavity, as shown in Figure 1.2.

The uterus is the site where a fertilized egg implants and develops into a baby. This remarkable organ gradually grows to accommodate the baby (or babies!) along with the placenta and amniotic fluid. With the onset of labor, the muscular contractions of the uterus forcibly dilate the cervix to push out the baby (with lots of help from the mother).

The inner lining of the uterus, the endometrium, thickens in response to estrogen and progesterone each month in preparation for pregnancy. This lining is shed as a menstrual period if pregnancy doesn't occur.

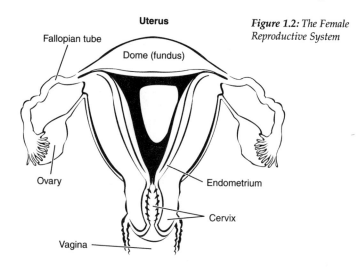

Figure 1.2: The Female Reproductive System

Cervix

The cervix is the entrance into the uterus from the vagina. This lower-most part of the uterus contains glands that secrete a watery mucus at the time of ovulation to help sperm get into the uterus for fertilization. During labor, the cervix must thin and dilate to allow a baby to be delivered.

The cervix is infamous for its propensity for developing cancer if left unchecked. A relatively simple and reliable test for pre-cancerous changes of the cervix is the Pap smear. This single test has greatly reduced the incidence of cervical cancer and saved many thousands of lives since its introduction.

Fallopian Tubes

The delicate fallopian tubes are connected to the uterus on one end and open to the ovaries on the other. They provide a passageway for fertilized eggs to reach the uterus. Conception (joining of egg and sperm) takes place at the far end of the tube, which is called the ampulla. The fertilized egg waits for a few days before migrating down the tube to implant in the uterus.

The fallopian tubes can be badly damaged by pelvic infections like gonorrhea or chlamydia, increasing the risk of tubal, or ectopic, pregnancy. If the tubes are destroyed, sterility will result. "Tying the tubes" refers to the intentional sterilization of a woman by using one of many techniques to permanently obstruct the fallopian tubes.

Ovaries

Measuring just longer than an inch, these tiny powerhouses produce the hormones that account for female body characteristics and physiology: estrogen and progesterone. Cell receptors (complex molecules with specific sensitivity to certain hormones) within the ovaries allow chemical communication with the brain as part of the menstrual cycle.

The ovaries release an egg for fertilization each month during a woman's reproductive years. The primary mechanism by which birth control pills work is by inhibiting the development and release of these eggs.

THE MENSTRUAL CYCLE

In the normal reproductive-aged female, the regular cyclic release of hormones from the brain and the ovaries results in the maturation and release of an egg every 28 days. When an egg is released at midcycle, it is picked up by a fallopian tube to await fertilization. At the same time, estrogen and progesterone, the primary ovarian hormones, stimulate the uterus to prepare it for pregnancy. If fertilization doesn't occur, a menstrual period results and the cycle begins again.

Why Is the Cycle Length 28 Days?

No one is certain, but it's probably related to lunar cycles and their effect on the brain.

A normal cycle length for some women may be as little as 21 days (from the start of bleeding until the start of the next flow) or as many as 35 days; the average is 28 days.

What Is a "Period" Anyway?

The period, or menses, or menstrual flow, is the shedding of the unused lining of the uterine cavity, the endometrium, when an egg is not fertilized. There is great variation between women in the amount of menstrual flow at the end of each cycle. Note also that not all vaginal bleeding represents a menstrual period. Bleeding can be caused by hormonal, infectious, precancerous/cancerous, or traumatic conditions of the vagina, cervix, or uterus.

What Are Estrogen and Progesterone?

Estrogen and progesterone are hormones, chemicals released in one part of the body that travel (usually via the bloodstream) to another part of the body to have their effects. Estrogen and progesterone are made by the ovaries in response to other hormones (FSH and LH) secreted by the pituitary gland in the brain. Their primary purpose is to ready the inner lining of the uterus for implantation of the fertilized egg, but they also influence the breasts and give feedback to the brain. This feedback is a chemical message to the pituitary that the ovaries have responded.

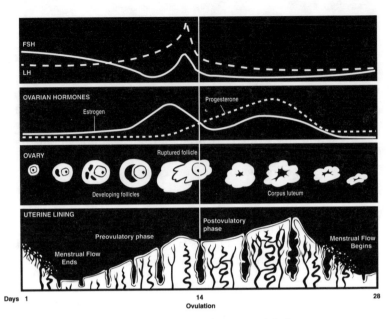

Figure 1.3: The Phases of the Menstrual Cycle

Estrogen is the hormone primarily responsible for breast development and other body changes in girls at puberty. Its decline at menopause causes the symptoms associated with that time of life, such as vaginal dryness and hot flashes.

Figure 1.3 shows the fluctuations of estrogen and progesterone along with the pituitary hormones FSH and LH, during a normal 28-day menstrual cycle. The cycle is divided into follicular and luteal phases. The follicular phase refers to the early part of the cycle, when the egg is maturing within the ovarian follicle; in the luteal phase, the corpus luteum of the ovary makes progesterone to mature the endometrial lining of the uterus. Ovulation occurs between the two phases.

When Is My Partner Fertile Each Month?

Your partner can become pregnant only during the 24 to 48 hours following ovulation (at midcycle, when the ovary releases a mature egg), which is approximately 14 days before the start of her next menstrual flow.

Do Men Have a Similar Hormonal Cycle?

No.

When Do Menstrual Cycles Start, and When Do They End?

On average, girls begin menstruating at around age 12 or 13, when the brain, ovaries, and adrenal glands are ready (the adrenal glands make hormones that promote early physical changes of puberty). Initial cycles are usually irregular and unpredictable because the hormonal communications are erratic. Pregnancy can occur just before a young girl's first menstrual period if she has already ovulated.

The average age for a woman to end her menstrual cycles (menopause) is 51. There is wide variation in this age, and the best predictor is the age at which the other women in her family (mother, sisters, etc.) stopped menstruating. Fertility declines rapidly from age 40, and effectively ends a couple of years before menopause.

Why Are Some Women Irregular or Without Periods Altogether?

There are many causes for absent or irregular cycles, such as thyroid gland dysfunction, excessive exercise or stress, or premature failure of the ovaries. Some women come from families with irregular, infrequent menstrual bleeding that is caused by an inherited defect in the hormonal cycle. This results in only intermittent ovulation.

The menstrual cycle can be intentionally interrupted by birth control pills or other hormonal treatments (medications like Depo-Provera or Gn-RH agonists) for the purpose of contraception and/or disease management. These medications work primarily by suppressing the release of the pituitary hormones that stimulate the ovaries. These interruptions are temporary, and the cycles typically return just after discontinuation of the treatment.

When menstrual cycles are erratic or absent in a woman not on these medications, it is appropriate to have a physician

investigate to determine the cause. Sometimes an easily cor-
rectable problem exists, such as an inactive thyroid gland;
treatment of this condition will not only restore the cycles, but
also may have other positive effects throughout the body.
Several other causes for irregular or absent cycles exist, and it's
important to determine the specific cause because of the potential long-term effects on health and fertility. A woman should
be aware of her diagnosis if she has irregular cycles.

What's the Brain Got to Do with It?

As mentioned above, the ovaries function in response to
hormonal commands (FSH and LH) from the pituitary. The
pituitary is in chemical communication with the hypothala-
mus, right above it. This delicate partnership is influenced by
numerous inputs from other centers within the brain, as well
as by the feedback information given by ovarian production of
estrogen and progesterone. Without these signals, the ovaries
would never mature and release an egg or make the hormones
that ready the uterine lining for pregnancy. Certain fertility
drugs, such as clomiphene citrate, work in the brain to
overcome problems with ovulation.

POST TEST

1. Most men have extensive knowledge about female anatomy.

   T or F

2. The cervix is actually a part of the uterus.

   T or F

3. Fallopian tubes are delicate structures that can be damaged by infections like chlamydia.

   T or F

4. The tube that empties the urinary bladder, the urethra, is much shorter in women than in men.

   T or F

5. All women have 28-day intervals from the start of one menstrual period to the start of another.

   T or F

6. The brain and the ovaries work together to control menstrual cycles.

   T or F

7. A menstrual period results from sloughing off of the unused lining of the uterus, the endometrium.

   T or F

8. Women will reach menopause, on average, at the age of 51.

   T or F

9. Estrogen and progesterone are hormones secreted by the pituitary gland in the brain.

   T or F

10. Pap smears are recommended at regular intervals to help detect early ovarian cancer.

    T or F

Key: 1. F 2. T 3. T 4. T 5. F 6. T 7. T 8. T 9. F 10. F

LET'S TALK ABOUT SEX, BABY   **2**

He was probably thinking about it, too.

Sex. Sex, sex, sex, sex, sex. And, oh yeah, sex.

For some men, this is an all-consuming interest—a "passion" in the truest sense of the word. In between thinking about, engaging in, or resting up after sex, they wedge in less important activities, like earning a living, eating, and doing an occasional wash.

Most men, thankfully, are more balanced in their approach toward sex. Like pearl divers holding their breath, some can go several minutes without even thinking about it. This, of course, takes years of practice and determination, and is not for everyone.

So, we think it's safe to say, and we're certainly not the first to say it, that sex is on men's minds. This being said, we realize it's probably not news to you or to anyone else. We can blame it on biology, we can say "It's the fault of (whatever group or individual it is currently stylish to blame for society's troubles)!" but it doesn't look like it's going to change any time soon.

Despite this passion, this obsession with sex, many guys lack basic knowledge about it. For instance, they don't know how to protect a woman from getting pregnant! And we don't have to tell you that unwanted pregnancy is a very serious issue in any relationship.

Therefore, in an effort to be helpful to our fellow men, we provide here a comprehensive guy's guide to **contraception**. In the pages that follow, you can read about the method you and your partner are now using, how it works, and any shortcomings it may have. And since contraceptive needs change over time, you should also check out the other available methods.

Just how impressed would your partner be if you became well informed about your birth control method? Who knows, you might even find a *better* method for the two of you. A lofty goal, perhaps, but we think you can do it.

Another area that guys could pay more attention to is known in medical circles as **female sexual response**. We tap into this body of knowledge and answer the following questions: What are the stages of sexual response? What happens to a woman's body as she becomes aroused? What sorts of things can interfere with her excitement? We even include some hints from a woman's perspective on what works to excite the female of the species.

We invite you to explore this brief dialogue. Perhaps you'll find some of this information helpful, despite your tremendous natural abilities when it comes to lovemaking.

(See? You're thinking about sex again.)

GUY-Q TEST

1. IUDs prevent pregnancy by:
   a. blocking the entrance to the cervix.
   b. preventing sperm from reaching the egg.
   c. disrupting the endometrial (uterus) lining, making it inhospitable for pregnancy.
   d. b and c.

2. Condoms, diaphragms, and cervical caps differ from hormonal methods of birth control (birth control pills, Depo-Provera) in which of the following ways?
   a. They are generally less effective at preventing pregnancy.
   b. They must be placed or inserted just prior to making love.
   c. They don't contain hormones.
   d. All of the above.

3. IUDs are:
   a. a cause of uterine cancer.
   b. a highly effective birth control device.
   c. previously the focus of a large class-action lawsuit.
   d. b and c.

4. True statements about birth control pills include:
   a. Forgetting to take pills each day greatly increases the chance of becoming pregnant.
   b. They can be used as emergency contraception when specially prescribed.
   c. When used for more than a year, they lower the risk of cancer of the uterus and ovaries.
   d. All of the above.

5. Condoms:
   a. must be placed on the penis *before* insertion into the vagina to be effective.
   b. should be lubricated with petroleum jelly before each use.
   c. can be used for multiple acts of intercourse.

6. Emergency contraception methods include:
   a. douching.
   b. IUD insertion.
   c. oral contraceptives.
   d. b and c.

7. Male sterilization:
   a. is routinely accomplished by removal of the testes.
   b. is irreversible.
   c. removes the sperm from the ejaculate fluid produced during orgasm.

8. Female orgasm is:
   a. affected by external, nonsexual factors.
   b. the result of appropriate stimulation of the female genitalia.
   c. characterized by rhythmic contractions of the uterus.
   d. all of the above.

9. The three stages of *female* sexual response are:
   a. interest, excitement, and climax.
   b. desire, arousal, and orgasm.

10. The three stages of *male* sexual response are:
    a. desire, arousal, and orgasm.
    b. desire, arousal, and "Oops, I thought you were ready."

Key: 1. d   2. d   3. d   4. d   5. a   6. d   7. c   8. d   9. b   10. a

CONTRACEPTION

Asked why he was calling with questions about his wife's birth control pill prescription:

"It just comes from caring about your spouse."

—Aaron B., Los Angeles, CA

"Birth control is more of a couple's issue than a woman's responsibility."

—Marianne M., Dana Point, CA

If there was ever a topic in gynecology that invited the participation of men, contraception is it. It surprises us that we don't see more men accompanying their partners to the office when we discuss contraception. The choice of birth control method will have a significant impact on a couple's sexual relationship, their chances for conceiving a child, and the risk of passage of sexually transmitted diseases (STDs) from one to the other.

Birth control is a complex subject, even for gynecologists. When we prescribe contraceptive methods, we have to consider for each patient a method's effectiveness, acceptability, cost, and safety, and its effectiveness in prohibiting the transmittal of STDs. As a woman's life changes, so do her needs in birth control. She may have started a new relationship, making protection from STDs more important. If she develops a health problem, it may require a change in method (for example, high blood pressure may make using birth control pills unwise). Her insurance may have changed, making cost a factor. A busy life may make it hard for her to remember to use her contraceptive, so she may need to change to a method that requires less conscious effort on her part.

What Are the Different Types of Birth Control?

For ease of understanding, we have divided the most commonly used birth control methods into the following categories, based on how they work:

- **Barrier methods**   Condoms, diaphragms, cervical caps, "the sponge," spermicidal foams/suppositories/creams/jellies
- **Hormonal methods**   Birth control pills, the minipill, the morning-after pill, Depo-Provera, Norplant
- **Other methods**   IUDs, sterilization, natural family planning, new methods.

We recommend that you read about *all* of the methods. You may learn something new about the method you're currently using, and you may also find that your present method isn't the best for your current situation. It is preferable for both members of a couple to participate in the choice and consistent use of a birth control method.

Barrier Methods

How Do Barrier Methods Work?

Barrier methods represent the earliest type of birth control devised. They are called barrier methods because they work by physically blocking the sperm from entering the cervix and upper genital tract, where the egg waits to be fertilized. Aside from contraception, they have the additional benefit of inhibiting the spread of many STDs by the same barrier action. Spermicides (chemicals used to inhibit sperm) may add further protection against pregnancy and disease. In particular, condoms are useful for protecting women at risk for acquiring infections.

One of the primary disadvantages of barrier methods is that they often require the user to apply them during foreplay—a time when logic and clear thinking are in short supply. This is a major reason why contraceptive failures (unintended pregnancies) with barrier methods are more common than with other methods.

Condoms

When used correctly, condoms are 90 to 98% effective; the best rates occur if a spermicide is used in conjuction with the condom. The bad news is that condoms are rarely used correctly every time, so actual effectiveness is considerably lower. Confusion about correct condom use contributes greatly to failure in preventing pregnancy.

The most common problems with condoms are from breakage, early removal or "slipping off," and lack of consistent use. Many men don't like the loss of sensation that may occur with condoms. As mentioned, the use of condoms requires interruption of foreplay, which greatly reduces the chances they'll be used every time.

The following suggestions on the proper use of condoms come from the Centers for Disease Control and Prevention (the recommendations are printed in their entirety at the end of Chapter 4):

- Use a new, latex condom for each act of intercourse.
- Open the condom package carefully and roll the condom all the way down the erect penis. Do this *before* intercourse.
- Leave space at the tip of the condom for semen (many condoms have "receptacle" tips).
- If you need more lubrication, use only water-based lubricants (ask a pharmacist). Oil-based lubricants (hand lotion, petroleum jelly, or baby oil) may weaken the condom.
- Withdraw from your partner while your penis is still erect, and hold on to the condom to keep it from slipping off.
- If you think the condom has broken, withdraw from your partner and put on a new one *immediately*.

If condoms are your sole method of birth control, use them correctly *every time.*

Diaphragms

A diaphragm is a latex ring (two to three inches across), which is placed inside the vagina to cover the cervix during intercourse.

Spermicide is used with the diaphragm, and the combination prevents sperm from passing into the upper genital tract.

Similar in effectiveness to condoms, the diaphragm prevents unwanted pregnancy 81 to 98% of the time. Like condoms, they are difficult to use effectively every time because they require user motivation during foreplay. Another disadvantage of this method is that it requires a visit to the doctor's office for fitting. Like condoms, the diaphragm must be in place before each act of intercourse in order to be effective.

One common side effect women experience with diaphragms is an increase in bladder infections. This may be caused by incomplete emptying of the bladder when the diaphragm is in place. As mentioned, the diaphragm may require couples to stop foreplay to use the method, but it *can* be inserted up to six hours before intercourse. On the plus side, diaphragm users have a lower incidence of gonorrhea, tubal infections, infertility, and precancer of the cervix than nonusers.

For best results with a diaphragm:

- Always use spermicide. Refresh the supply within the vagina before each act of intercourse.
- Leave the diaphragm in place in the vagina for at least six hours after intercourse, but no more than 24 hours.
- Replace the diaphragm with a new one every year or so. Hold it up to a light (not too close) to check it for holes once a month.

When you and your mate are using the diaphragm or any of the barrier methods, remember: They must be used correctly *each time* to be effective. Help your partner remember to use it!

Cervical Cap

Similar to the diaphragm, the cervical cap covers the cervix to prevent sperm passage. It is smaller than a diaphragm and fits snugly over the cervix when properly applied. Its effectiveness is in the 88 to 98% range when used correctly.

Drawbacks to this method are that the cervical cap is more difficult to insert because of its smaller size and it may *increase* the risk of cervical precancer. It also cannot be used near the time of menstrual bleeding because of the risk of toxic shock syndrome, a serious bacterial infection.

Recommendations for cervical cap use are similar to those for the diaphragm:

- Keep the cervical cap in place for eight hours after intercourse.
- Spermicide is only necessary if STD protection is a concern.

Help her remember! Did we mention, help her remember?

Contraceptive Sponge, Vaginal Foams/Creams/Jellies, and Suppositories

Spermicides work by forming a chemical barrier to the passage of sperm. The chemical is usually nonoxynol-9, a potent spermicide that disables or kills sperm on contact. Somewhat less effective than other options, spermicide use alone results in unwanted pregnancy in up to 26% of couples in a year's use.

The problems with chemical barrier methods are that they are somewhat messy to use and are often used incorrectly. Contraceptive sponge users also run a higher risk of toxic shock syndrome if a woman is menstruating, or if the sponge is left in place for more than 24 hours.

It is important to know that nonoxynol-9 is not associated with birth defects if a woman becomes pregnant while using it.

For best results with these methods:

- Apply the spermicide *just before* intercourse.
- Use a condom, diaphragm, or cervical cap in combination with the spermicide to significantly improve contraceptive effectiveness.

Help her remember! You're in this together!

Hormonal Methods

How Do Hormonal Methods Work?

As you learned in Chapter 1, a woman conceives a pregnancy when she produces an egg (ovulation) and it is penetrated by a sperm (fertilization) in her fallopian tube. This process of egg maturation and release and the successful implantation of the fertilized egg in the uterus is dependent on the orderly release of estrogen and progesterone during a woman's menstrual cycle. Hormonal contraception alters a woman's menstrual cycle to achieve some or all of the following: prevention of ovulation, prevention of fertilization through a thickening of the cervical mucus, and prevention of implantation by rendering the lining of the uterus inhospitable for pregnancy.

Some of the hormonal methods of birth control have noncontraceptive health benefits. In addition, they do not require interruption of foreplay for their use and are therefore more likely to be used consistently.

Both oral contraceptives and Norplant may not work as well if a woman is also using certain antibiotics or seizure medications. If she is prescribed one of these medications, it is best to discuss this with her doctor.

The most significant limitation of hormonal contraceptives is that they do not provide any protection against HIV and other STDs.

In any new or nonmonogamous relationship, the use of condoms along with effective hormonal contraception is a good idea for both partners.

Oral Contraceptives

Modern oral contraceptive pills (OCs) contain both a synthetic estrogen and a synthetic progesterone in doses sufficient to prevent ovulation. They do this by inhibiting the release of pituitary hormones that stimulate the ovaries. OCs also make the cervical mucus somewhat thicker, which helps to block sperm passage into the uterus and tubes. When used properly, this method carries a 98 to 99% success rate in preventing pregnancy.

Perhaps the most difficult aspect of using OCs for contraception is that it requires the woman to take them every single day. Frequently forgetting to take pills raises the risk of pregnancy significantly. If a woman misses a pill, she should take two pills the next day. If she misses two or more pills in a row, she should take two pills a day until she catches up; she should also use a backup method of contraception (condoms or a diaphragm) until her period comes.

Standard low-dose pills today are of two types. Monophasic pills have constant doses of estrogen and progesterone throughout the menstrual cycle; examples are Ovcon-35 and Ortho-Novum 1/35. Triphasic pills (Tri-Norinyl, Ortho-Novum 7/7/7) have stable estrogen levels, but the progesterone component varies throughout the cycle. These triphasic pills have a slightly lower total dose of progesterone, which may decrease the occurrence and severity of side effects.

What Are the More Common Side Effects of the Pill?

Side effects of OCs have long been a concern to users and often account for the decision to switch to a different method. Today's birth control pills contain significantly less hormone than their predecessors and have fewer side effects. Many of the more common complaints resolve after the first one to three months of use. Typical early complaints are nausea, breast tenderness, and "breakthrough" bleeding (bleeding during the middle of the pack of pills instead of at the end). Some of the other more common side effects include:

- **Weight gain** The amount of weight gain attributable to the pill is believed to be no more than 2 to 3 pounds. One study showed that women on OCs were as likely to gain weight over time as a similar group who were not taking them.

- **Absent menstrual periods** The regular bleeding seen at the end of the pack of pills in most women may not be present in some. The *only* value of bleeding in women on OCs is that it indicates that they are not pregnant. Absent bleeding in a woman taking the pill reliably and without symptoms of pregnancy (breast tenderness, nausea) may be acceptable. Lighter menstrual bleeding on OCs is one of the major advantages of the pill.

- **Headaches** Tension headaches are no more common for women on OCs than for those not taking them. If migraine headaches become more frequent or severe, the pill may have to be stopped because of a slightly increased risk of stroke.

- **PMS (premenstrual syndrome)/depression/mood swings** These side effects are seen in some women on OCs. Interestingly, many women notice a significant improvement in PMS while on the pill.

- **Decreased breast milk production** Occasionally, women may notice trouble with breast-feeding after delivery when restarting the pill.

Women who experience side effects are encouraged to contact their health care providers before abandoning their pills. Often, dietary changes, switching to a different pill, or the passage of time will resolve their complaints.

Are There Any Serious Health Risks from Taking the Pill?

Serious health concerns about the safety of OCs were raised after the first decade of their use. With careful scientific analysis and evaluation of the new, lower-dose pills, the following conclusions were reached:

- **Risks in pregnancy** Fears of birth defects have largely disappeared. OCs do not cause *any* effects on the fetus if stopped before the ninth week of pregnancy.

- **Increased risk of heart attack/stroke** Only if the woman is over 35 and smokes cigarettes (21 times higher risk if she smokes three-quarters of a pack or more per day!) or has other risk factors (severe migraines, high cholesterol) will the pill increase her risk of heart attack or stroke.

- **Increased risk of gallbladder disease** Women on the pill will experience a small increased risk of gallstones, primarily in those predisposed to this disorder.

- **Elevated blood pressure** Mild increases in blood pressure are noted in rare cases. All women should have their blood pressure checked after beginning OCs to make sure it hasn't increased. Low-dose OCs may now be safely prescribed for some patients with well-controlled, mild high blood pressure.

- **Liver cancer** There is no increased risk; however, benign (noncancerous) tumors rarely occur in women on low-dose OCs.

- **Altered blood sugar (carbohydrate) metabolism** This is rare with low-dose OCs. The newer pills can even be used by diabetics whose disease is well controlled.

- **Infertility** The pill does not cause infertility. However, a woman who has been on the pill may need longer to conceive after discontinuing the OC (fertility rates are the same after one year).

There is no overall increased risk of breast cancer in women 20 to 54 who have taken OCs.

Does Taking the Pill Have Any Health Benefits?

Initial concerns about side effects and health risks damaged the pill's reputation as a safe method of contraception. In a poll conducted for the American College of Obstetricians and Gynecologists in 1985, 75% of women believed that taking birth control pills carried substantial health risks. In light of the information presented above, this public opinion has begun to change. In addition to the fact that many of the health risks of OCs were overestimated, it's important to know that there are substantial health benefits for most women from taking OCs:

- fewer benign breast cysts, which often require surgery for removal;

- lighter, more predictable menstrual periods;

- less pain with menstrual periods (cramps);

- lower rates of pelvic inflammatory disease (PID);

- 50% lower rate of cancer of the uterine lining (endometrial cancer) after one year on OCs;

- 40–80% decrease in risk of ovarian cancer, depending on the number of years of OC use;

- lower risk of tubal (ectopic) pregnancies.

Women in their 30s and 40s now commonly take birth control pills for the noncontraceptive benefits they offer. Most healthy women at any age before menopause may start OCs and use them for an unlimited period. The majority of women tolerate oral contraceptives well and derive numerous health benefits as well as excellent contraception from taking them.

If your partner stops taking the pill, she must start a new method *immediately*. Many unintended pregnancies occur just after couples stop OCs.

The Minipill

The minipill (trade name Micronor) is so named because it contains progesterone only. Because there is no estrogen component, some of the common side effects of the pill (nausea, headaches) are less likely. Unfortunately, the lack of estrogen also causes some side effects, chiefly irregular, unpredictable bleeding. Ovulation is also incompletely inhibited, which causes this method to be less effective than OCs that contain both progesterone and estrogen: 92 to 95%. The minipill is most commonly given to women who cannot tolerate estrogen side effects and can't use other methods. The minipill is also popular with breast-feeding women because regular birth control pills may decrease breast milk production.

The Morning-After Pill

Not a method recommended for routine use, this hormonal contraceptive was created for use in emergency situations (such as a broken condom). The contraceptive effect is achieved by inhibiting ovulation, as well as chemically altering the endometrium (uterine lining). This is accomplished by taking two high-dose OCs and repeating the dosage twelve hours later, within 72 hours of intercourse. Nausea and vomiting are common side effects. When used properly, the method is fairly effective (75%) in preventing pregnancy.

A recent study conducted at Princeton University examined students' perceptions of the morning-after pill. Only a quarter of those interviewed were aware that it is only about 75% effective. Thirty-seven percent of the students interviewed believed that the medication was 100% effective in preventing pregnancy. The researchers concluded that more education about this method was needed.

C. C. Harper and C. E. Euerston, "The emergency contraceptive pill: A study of knowledge and attitudes among students at Princeton University," *American Journal of Obstetrics and Gynecology* 173(5): 1438 (1995).

Depo-Provera

Despite its recent appearance in the United States, Depo-Provera (also known as Depo-Medroxyprogesterone Acetate) is far from new. Used by more than 11 million women in 80 countries for more than 20 years, Depo-Provera is a highly effective contraceptive with a long track record.

Like the minipill, Depo-Provera is a progesterone-only method. The synthetic progesterone is given as an intra-muscular injection every three months. High circulating levels of progesterone in the blood suppress ovulation, thicken cervical mucus, and prevent implantation of fertilized eggs by altering the lining of the uterus. These effects result in a pregnancy rate of less than one percent of couples using the method.

The drug company that markets this product proclaims this is birth control "you only have to think about four times a year" (because each injection lasts three months). This infrequent interval does help women to continue with the method, but there is a drawback: any side effects may also last a full three months.

What Side Effects Can Occur with Depo-Provera?

Some of the more common complaints from Depo-Provera users are:

• **Weight gain**   Average weight gain in the first year is five pounds, three pounds in the second year.

• **Mood changes**   A small percentage of patients experience nervousness, decreased sex drive, or depression.

• **Delayed return to normal fertility**   Like OCs, Depo-Provera doesn't cause infertility. However, it may take couples longer to conceive after its use is discontinued (studies show that the average time to conception is 10 months).

• **Breakthrough bleeding**   Twenty to thirty percent of women using Depo-Provera will have irregular unpredictable bleeding while on the medication. This is the largest single reason for discontinuation of Depo-Provera.

• **Lack of menstrual bleeding**   A common side effect is lack of menstrual bleeding. Fifty percent of women will stop having periods after one year of use. This is not a permanent effect—menstrual periods will resume after stopping Depo-Provera.

- **Decreased bone density** Decreased bone density is a possible effect over time with Depo-Provera. At present, the loss appears insignificant, and it disappears after the woman stops using the medicine.

For many women, these side effects don't pose much of a problem. The weight gain is usually mild, significant mood changes are unusual, and most couples don't mind a brief decline in their fertility after discontinuing Depo-Provera. The irregular bleeding is a nuisance, but the total volume of blood loss per month is less than a normal period. Finally, many women appreciate the temporary absence of bleeding and not having to think about birth control very often. According to the World Health Organization, there is no increased risk of cancer of the uterus, ovaries, breasts, or cervix from using Depo-Provera.

What Health Benefits Are Found with Depo-Provera?

The following noncontraceptive health benefits occur with Depo-Provera:

- less endometrial (uterine lining) cancer;
- lighter, less painful periods;
- symptoms of PMS may be improved.

If she's using Depo-Provera, remind her to get her injection *on time* every three months.

Norplant

Another progesterone-only hormonal method, Norplant works by releasing a synthetic progesterone compound into the bloodstream through six small capsules "planted" under the skin of the upper arm. This birth control method lasts for five years, and once inserted has a 97 to 99% effectiveness rating in preventing pregnancy. Its "mechanism of action" is similar to the other hormonal methods; the progesterone inhibits ovulation, thickens cervical mucus, or alters the endometrial lining to prevent implantation.

One significant drawback to Norplant is that it requires an in-office minor surgical procedure to place or remove the capsules. There is very little pain or risk associated with the procedures, but it is a definite drawback in most women's minds. Insertion of the capsules takes about 10 minutes. Removal may take 30 minutes or more because of the fibrosis (scarring) that forms around the capsules. No large scars should result when the removal is done correctly.

Another complaint is purely cosmetic: the capsules can often be seen just under the skin of the arm.

What Side Effects Occur with Norplant?

- **Irregular bleeding**   Irregular and unpredictable bleeding is the biggest complaint of users. Typically the bleeding becomes less of a problem after the first year.
- **Weight gain**   Weight gain in women using Norplant is similar to the other hormonal methods.
- **Headaches**   Headaches while using Norplant are usually a temporary problem.
- **Mood changes**   Depression is seen occasionally.

What Health Benefits Occur with Norplant Use?

Benefits of Norplant include its long-term effectiveness (five years) and ease of use: once the capsules are inserted, Norplant requires *no effort* on the part of the user to be effective. Fertility also returns promptly once the capsules are removed.

Thorough counseling by health care professionals is important *before* the insertion of Norplant. Both partners should understand the side effects, risks, and benefits of this method in detail (as you should for all methods!).

Our patients seem to appreciate it when their partners accompany them to their insertion or removal appointments.

Other Methods

Intrauterine Devices (IUDs)

The IUD, a small twisted plastic device scarcely three inches long, is placed in a woman's uterine cavity. Following the insertion, a woman is virtually incapable of becoming pregnant. No hormones are altered within her bloodstream, no visible devices are worn or felt by either partner; she never has to *think* about contraception once the device is inserted. Sound too good to be true? Well, for many women it is true, but the modern IUD came to us on a road as twisted as the contraceptive itself.

Intrauterine devices were a very popular method of contraception when they were introduced in the 1970s. They provided excellent effectiveness (95–98%) immediately after a simple in-office placement procedure. There were relatively few side effects compared to the available contraceptive methods of the time, and the device required almost no attention once it was inserted. Many women in many different circumstances (single, married, teens, and moms) used them.

Coincidentally, the 1970s also saw the continuation of the "free love" movement, and, to put it bluntly, a lot of people slept with a lot of other people, who were sleeping with any number of other people, some of whom they knew. As the decade wore on, the medical community witnessed a connection between IUD use and pelvic inflammatory disease (PID), a bacterial infection caused by gonorrhea and/or chlamydia. PID is serious because it increases the risk of infertility, ectopic pregnancy, and chronic pain.

It was finally shown that IUD use promoted the development of PID in two ways: The IUD insertion procedure could carry bacteria into the uterine cavity, and the string of one particular IUD also promoted infection. The Dalkon Shield became infamous because it had a multifilament string that quite efficiently transported vaginal bacteria into the sterile confines of the uterus.

As the association between IUDs and PID reached the medical community, responsible physicians began to withdraw their recommendation of the IUD. Attorneys sought to win large awards against the physicians and manufacturers who, in the majority, had not knowingly done anything wrong in previously prescribing the IUD. Many of these lawsuits were successful for the plaintiffs. Not surprisingly, this method of contraception disappeared as quickly and completely as did Jimmy Hoffa.

Battered and bruised, the IUD has bravely reappeared in recent years. To protect itself in these dangerously litigious times, it returned with a rather lengthy informed consent statement that patients must sign before insertion. One gets the feeling when reading this consent statement that if a woman suffered a complication while using an IUD, the pharmaceutical company could sue *her*.

Is There More Than One Type of IUD?

There are currently two IUDs available in the U.S: the Progestasert and the Paraguard. The Progestasert contains a small amount of synthetic progesterone, which has a local contraceptive effect on the uterine lining. It is effective for one year from insertion. The Paraguard has thin copper wire wrapped around the plastic arms, which enhances its contraceptive effect. Once placed, it lasts for ten years. Both IUDs contain a short mono-filament string that hangs out of the cervix to allow women to verify that the IUD is still present and in the proper location.

How Does an IUD Prevent Pregnancy?

According to the World Health Organization, the IUD works primarily by inhibiting fertilization: Local effects from the IUD within the uterus are unfavorable to sperm activity. This is important information for couples who are opposed to abortion of any kind. However, inflammatory changes caused by the IUD within the uterus are also inhospitable to implantation of an embryo, if conception does occur. This makes the IUD useful as an emergency contraceptive in some cases. The device is usually placed while a woman is having her period, but it can be placed at any time as long as she is not pregnant.

What Side Effects Occur with IUD Use?

- **Increased menstrual bleeding** Most women notice some increase in menstrual flow while the IUD is in place.

- **More menstrual pain, or cramps** The mild local inflammation caused by the IUD often results in slightly more severe menstrual cramps. The pain is usually well managed with antiprostaglandin medications, such as Advil or Motrin.

- **Penile irritation** If the string on the end of the IUD is left too long, it can poke the end of the penis during sex. This is a simple problem to correct, requiring just a brief office visit to trim the string.

Are There Serious Risks with IUD Use?

Complications can still occur with IUD use, so patients must be aware of what to look for:

- **IUD expulsion** The device can be expelled from the uterus during heavy menstrual flow, and sometimes this can go unnoticed. Users should check for the string each month to verify that the IUD is in place.

- **Perforation of the uterus** The IUD can escape into the pelvic cavity if a hole is made in the wall of the uterus. This generally happens during insertion. When perforation occurs, the contraceptive effect is lost immediately. Checking for the string each month will confirm this hasn't occurred. Surgery may be required to retrieve the IUD because of a small risk of bowel injury if the device is left in the pelvis.

- **Pelvic inflammatory disease** The risk of PID is still increased with IUD use, but occurs only if a woman is exposed to gonorrhea or chlamydia. Antibiotics are sometimes given at the time of insertion to reduce the risk. Studies show that the risk is increased only for the first one to four months after insertion. Because of the potential complications after an episode of PID, we don't usually recommend the IUD for women who have more than one sexual partner or who have not completed their families.

- **Miscarriage with/without infection** A three-times higher rate of miscarriage occurs if a woman conceives with an IUD in place. Since IUDs provide excellent contraception, this is very uncommon. If a woman does get pregnant with an IUD, we must also watch out for infection. No problems with birth defects are seen because of the IUD.

On balance, the benefits of the IUD are substantial for the right woman. The IUD is very convenient, requiring only a moment each month to verify its position. The method is extremely effective in preventing unwanted pregnancy and has no hormonal side effects. Finally, the copper IUD lasts for 10 years.

If she uses an IUD, remind her to check the string each month after her period.

Sterilization/Male

Many men fear loss of masculinity or castration in association with vasectomy. In reality, all that is entailed with this minor surgery is the occlusion (blockage) of the vas deferens, the duct that carries the sperm. The operation does not decrease testosterone output, and no removal of the testes (or any other structure) takes place.

Certain men are not candidates for this operation. Men with systemic blood disorders such as hemophilia, local infections of the genital tissues, or prior genital surgery that would make the surgery more difficult might be better off not having a vasectomy.

There are a few different methods used for vasectomy; a urologic surgeon can provide these details. Regardless of technique, once the vas is occluded, the ejaculate (fluid produced by the penis during orgasm) is soon devoid of sperm. Less than one in 100 guys has any detectable sperm after the operation, and this risk goes down significantly with time. Other minor complications such as bleeding and infection occur in less than five percent of surgeries.

Can a Vasectomy Be Undone?

Some men wish to have their vasectomies reversed because of remarriage, loss of children, change of mind, psychological reasons, or, rarely, recurrent pain or infections. In one large study of more than 1,000 men with such reversals, 86% had sperm present after the procedure.* Pregnancy resulted in a large percentage of these cases after the reversals. The best results were obtained in men who were within three years of their vasectomy. However, as with female sterilization, it is

*A. M. Belkar et al., "Results of 1,469 microsurgical vasectomy reversals by the vasovasostomy study group," *Journal of Urology* 145: 505 (1991).

best to be certain before going through with the surgery in the first place.

Another fear that has surfaced recently in the scientific community is that of prostate cancer after vasectomy. In 1991, the World Health Organization stated that testicular or prostate cancer is not likely to be related to vasectomy. At the present time, it is not possible to make a definitive statement, but most experts feel there might be "some increased risk" of prostate cancer in men who have had a vasectomy. Again, a urologic surgeon would be the best person to ask about this risk.

Research is inconclusive regarding the risk of kidney stones after vasectomy. There is, however, *no* increased risk of any systemic illness like cardiovascular disease. There is even some suggestion that overall death rates for men who have had a vasectomy are lower than for those who haven't.

This option, then, does deserve to be considered as a permanent means of birth control. Vasectomy has a better than 99% effectiveness rating, it can be accomplished through a very brief outpatient surgery, and its side effects and complications are comparable to female sterilization.

Sterilization/Female

Female sterilization is accomplished by blocking the fallopian tubes; this prevents sperm from getting to the egg. When done correctly, female sterilization is extremely effective at preventing pregnancy (98+%). The drawbacks of this method are that it requires a surgical procedure and is irreversible.

The most common techniques for female sterilization in the United States are to use suture, clips, or cautery (electrical current) to block the tubes in their midsection. Pregnancies occur after this surgery in one to two percent of cases, and these pregnancies may be caused by microscopic holes that develop in the remaining parts of the tube after they heal from the operation. Sperm are very tiny (and very determined), so they need only a tiny opening to exit the tube and find an egg to fertilize.

Are There Serious Risks After Sterilization?

A woman who becomes pregnant after a tubal sterilization runs a high risk of tubal or ectopic pregnancy. This is because the tube is already damaged by the sterilization surgery and the developing embryo often can't find its way to the uterus. Ectopic pregnancy is a very dangerous problem that can cause internal bleeding and even death.

Various clips and rings also have been devised to block the fallopian tubes. Their primary advantage is to offer the woman a slightly higher chance of reversing the sterilization if she changes her mind later on. Some physicians also find their application in surgery to be easier.

The sterilization operation can be performed at the same time as a cesarean section. It also can be done via laparoscopy as an outpatient; women can return to full function in a few days.

If your partner has had a tubal sterilization surgery and then develops symptoms of pregnancy at any time afterward, she should see her physician immediately to rule out a tubal pregnancy.

Natural Family Planning

Natural family planning relies on meticulous monitoring of a woman's body changes each month. Also known as the rhythm method, this method of birth control is often chosen for religious reasons.

As mentioned in Chapter 1, ovulation occurs 14 days before the menstrual flow begins in a normal menstrual cycle. The actual fertile period lasts for 24 to 48 hours after ovulation occurs. Certain predictable body changes occur at the time of ovulation, including an increase in the volume and water content of the cervical mucus and a slight increase in body temperature. Ovulation can usually be detected at the expected time in the month by noting (1) discomfort in the region of one of the ovaries, (2) an increase in watery vaginal discharge (from the cervical mucus), or (3) an increase in body temperature. By using these cues and keeping close track of menstrual cycle lengths, a woman can become more aware of her fertile times and prevent unwanted pregnancy.

Couples who use natural family planning avoid sex for several days each month before, during, and after their fertile period. Not surprisingly, natural family planning is not very popular nor effective enough for most couples. Every year, 20% of couples that rely on it will conceive a child.

Female Condoms

The female condom is a new contraceptive creation. A barrier method for women, it provides at least as much protection from pregnancy and STDs as does the male condom. Female condoms accomplish this by covering the vagina and labia (just outside the vagina), as well as the base of the penis.

Female condoms require no prescriptions or special fitting and can be inserted several hours before sex. Failure rates may exceed 20%, primarily because of improper use.

RU-486

RU-486 (also known as the French abortion pill) works by blocking the effects of circulating progesterone, which is necessary to establish and maintain pregnancy. RU-486 is used in Europe and Asia to induce abortions with a high degree of effectiveness and only mild side effects.

RU-486 is currently being studied in the United States for the treatment of uterine fibroids and other diseases. It is not available for contraceptive use.

New Contraceptive Developments

Copper IUDs may be inserted up to 10 days after unprotected intercourse to prevent implantation of an embryo. Initial studies show a very high effectiveness with this technique. It cannot be used in women at risk for STDs.

A new contraceptive gel that may also prevent STDs is being tested. In animals, it protects against herpes and prevents pregnancy. Transmission of HIV, gonorrhea, and chlamydia may also be blocked. The gel contains a chemical agent (methylcyanoacrylate) and will block the tubes from *inside* the uterus. The gel is inserted through the vagina without anesthesia and then into the near end of each fallopian tube. Preliminary results suggest a high rate of effectiveness.

A vaginal ring placed near the cervix is being studied. It would release estrogen and progesterone directly into the surrounding tissues.

Norplant may produce a two-capsule version (instead of six), designed for easier insertion and removal. However, its lifespan would be reduced as well.

New, nonlatex condoms are being tested and released. The new condoms are thinner, stronger, and less allergenic. If sensitivity is improved, it may lead to increased condom use.

A silicone barrier contraceptive designed to fit over the cervix may soon be available. It is designed to be more stable while in use, and may be particularly good for latex-sensitive individuals.

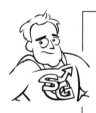

In conclusion, many different contraceptive methods are available. A method's effectiveness, safety, protection from disease, and ease of use should be considered. The best results will be obtained if *both* of you participate in the choice and consistent use of your birth control method. As we emphasize throughout *Your Guy's Guide to Gynecology*, your partner will appreciate your involvement.

FEMALE SEXUAL RESPONSE

"He just has a fascination with the female body. He's read books *about it."*

Has it made your sex life better?

"Yes! He knew what to do. He made me want *him."*

—A. J., San Diego, CA

Does it seem strange to you that men typically know very little about female sexual response? Given that most of us spend a significant amount of our early adult lives fantasizing about, desperately hoping for, and then finally acting out our fantasies of sexual fulfillment with a woman, doesn't it make sense that we would have researched this area at some time?

If you had wanted a Porsche for years, if you dreamed of racing it around a curve with your hair flying or just waxing it lovingly in your driveway, you'd likely spend some time learning about the car. Sure, you might hang pictures of a red Carrera with the black cloth roof in your locker, but you'd also keep back issues of *Car and Driver* around if they contained crucial articles on an extended road test or engine data. To put it bluntly, you'd *study* the car and do everything to maximize your pending relationship with it. You'd probably even *enjoy* the learning as a part of the whole experience.

So then, why is it that even the most enlightened new-age guys are mostly unaware of the physiologic functioning of women during sex? Although you don't need to be an expert, a little bit of knowledge about what is actually happening to your mate while you make love may make you a better lover. And if *she's* happier, guess who will be the primary recipient of her increased satisfaction? So read on, and then *apply* some of what you learn the next time you and she "speed down the highway of love."

What Are the Stages of Sexual Response?

Sexual response can be broken down into desire, arousal, and orgasm. Each person's sexual response is unique and is a function of past and present societal, familial, interpersonal, and personal experience.

Desire

Desire is the basic drive that results in the *willingness* to initiate or respond to sexual advances. This stage is more psychological than physical. Prior positive experiences reinforce desire; negative ones will diminish it.

What Sorts of Things Can Interfere with Her Excitement?

Situational factors such as distractions (crying babies, phone calls), physical pain from illness or injury, anger or dissatisfaction with a partner, substance abuse, or psychological problems (depression, history of sexual abuse) play an important role. Long-standing problems with arousal or orgasm also will eventually affect desire. All sorts of sexual and nonsexual issues in a relationship will either fan her flame or blow it out.

Certain medications can affect a woman's sex drive. Fluoxetine hydrochloride (trade name Prozac) and some other antidepressants can decrease it. They may also get in the way of a woman's ability to reach orgasm. Her doctor may recommend a "drug holiday" (taking a brief break from the medication) or changing to a different drug. Some antidepressants may cause an increased sex drive!

Other drugs known to affect libido are antihypertensives, anticonvulsants, antihistamines, and diuretics.

Arousal

This is where the fun starts. With a healthy amount of desire for further sexual intimacy on both parts, the stage is set for the preparatory physical activities that lead to orgasm. During this phase, you are using various parts of your body to stimulate and arouse your mate, primarily your hands, mouth, and finally your penis.

What Happens to a Woman's Body as She Becomes Excited?

As a woman becomes aroused, you may notice the following:

- **Breasts** Nipple erection; increase in breast size and dilation of blood vessels
- **Skin changes** A flush, or slight red rash, over the upper abdomen and breasts, spreading gradually

- **Muscle tension**   Voluntary tensing of abdominal and rib cage muscles

- **Heart**   Rate increases in response to rising tension; rates of 100–175 beats per minute on average

- **Blood pressure**   Elevations occur with rising tension

- **Clitoris**   Swells and elongates as the veins within it fill with blood

- **Vagina**   Lubrication; length and caliber of the vaginal canal increase; outer one-third of vagina swells, forming the "orgasmic platform"

- **Uterus**   Raises up; uterine body becomes increasingly sensitive to stimulation

- **Labia majora**   Slight lateral movement away from the vaginal opening; swelling from dilated veins

- **Labia minora**   Minor thickening and expansion; vivid color change to deep red as orgasm nears.

What's the Best Way to Excite a Woman?

As mentioned, the extent of these physical changes (her arousal) depends on the level of desire she started with and how skillfully her partner stimulates her. There is certainly no right way to arouse a woman, and you'll have to find your own road with your mate. What she prefers will probably also change over time as your relationship evolves. The following subtle suggestions were found in an article in *Men's Health* magazine (March 1995) by Jen Sacks, entitled "What Women Wish Men Knew about Sex":

- **Start here:** Just 15 minutes of foreplay. Kiss me like I'm the only thing in the world that exists right now. Please refrain from sticking your tongue all the way down my throat. Take your time . . . one serious kiss from a man gets me further than 20 minutes of attention to the more obvious places.

- **Make me comfortable:** Make sure your friends are out of the apartment first. If you happen to love me, say it.

- **Begin to touch me all over:** Gently, like it's something you've never seen before. Work your way up to things. Use your mouth. Everywhere. Let go of some of your inhibitions, but don't overwhelm me.

- **Give me a C. Give me an L. Give me an I-T-O-R-I-S.** What have you got? An almost sobbing, gently trembling, sometimes shouting right-out-loud woman. Go gently there, boys, whether it's your finger or another part of your body. By the way, good oral sex almost always works.

- **Make my day:** Some women do get there from vaginal intercourse alone. Try different positions until she tells you what works—or until it becomes obvious. Just pounding away, roughly or endlessly, does it for very few of us. As for *your* orgasm, what's often best for us is if you hold off as long as you can.

The bottom line here is to pay attention to her and how she is responding to your efforts. Be willing to adapt to your partner's needs, and don't forget to show affection and caring.

Orgasm

The third stage of the cycle occurs for the woman at the height of arousal with the surrender of control, and is characterized by certain physiologic events:

- **Muscles** Loss of voluntary control; contraction and spasm of muscle groups
- **Hyperventilation** Respiratory rate increases as high as 40/minute
- **Blood pressure/heart rate** Even greater increases than seen in the arousal phase
- **Vagina** Muscular contractions of the outer one-third of the vagina, 5–12 times, with gradual decline in intensity
- **Uterus** Contractions starting at the top of the uterus and progressing toward the cervix
- **Labia minora** Gradual decline in color change and venous congestion after orgasm

Are Men and Women the Same After an Orgasm?

Women can feel quite differently from men after an orgasm. They are often wide awake and eager for more, when their partners begin drifting off to sleep. Perhaps this capacity for multiple orgasm is compensation for having to endure the difficulties of menstrual periods and childbirth. As Jen Sacks put it, "Orgasm doesn't always end the arousal. Sometimes it leads to subsequent orgasms. Sometimes to insatiability." Understanding that this is a normal part of female sexual response and even anticipating it by not pulling away after your orgasm will increase your mate's pleasure.

What If Our Sexual Relationship Isn't Quite as Good as It Could Be?

We end this brief foray into the female sexual response with a note about sexual dysfunction. It quickly becomes clear when studying this topic that problems with sex in long-term relationships are quite common. Masters and Johnson, the noted sex researchers, estimated that 50% of married couples will have difficulties at some time.

A good physical relationship is very important to marital satisfaction; it is also quite vulnerable to disruption from factors within and outside of the relationship. Persistent problems with desire, arousal, or orgasm in either or both partners, regardless of their cause, need to be addressed. A competent physician or therapist with an interest in sexual therapy can often provide brief, symptom-focused treatment for couples that is highly effective.

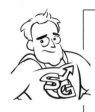

Supportive Guy Recommends:

- **Clean up your own act** Exercise regularly and lose weight if you need to.

- **Avoid boring sexual routine** Experiment with different locations and times of day in your love-making. Surprise her.

- **Keep distractions to a minimum** Don't allow interruptions to break the mood.

- **Be interested in her** Even when she talks about something you don't care about, you can show you care about *her*. Emotional intimacy increases the desire to be physically close.

- **Work on improving your relationship** Remember, desire is more psychological than physical. Respect her point of view, address problems directly, and work toward solutions (not toward being proved "right").

- **Don't be afraid to ask for help** If you find yourself wondering if your relationship needs some help in this area, it may be time to look into it. Gynecologists, therapists, and family doctors should know capable specialists near you.

POST TEST

1. The diaphragm is a good example of a hormonal method of birth control.

   T or F

2. Barrier methods work by blocking the entrance to the vagina.

   T or F

3. "I thought you were using something" is *not* an acceptable method of contraception.

   T or F

4. Birth control pills usually make a woman flow more heavily during her menstrual cycle.

   T or F

5. Birth control pills will lower the risk of cancer of the uterus and ovaries if used for a year or more.

   T or F

6. The IUD has a string on the end of it that allows a woman to check its location each month.

   T or F

7. Depo-Provera injections must be given once a year to be effective.

   T or F

8. Sexual desire can be greatly reduced for a woman if there are other problems in the relationship.

   T or F

9. Many women prefer slow, patient, and gentle stimulation as they become aroused.

   T or F

10. Women may remain excited after an orgasm and want more stimulation.

    T or F

Key: 1. F   2. F   3. T   4. F   5. T   6. T   7. F   8. T   9. T   10. T

VAGINITIS

3

We tried. We really tried. We wanted so much to make this an entertaining chapter, a story that just begged to be told on the big screen. But it wasn't to be. This just happens to be a fairly dry topic.

Vaginitis is certainly not funny to women who suffer from it. Think of how much you'd be laughing if you had penis-itis. You wouldn't want women laughing at your red, swollen, and sore love-muscle, would you? It's time for you to read some serious stuff to help your mate. So here goes, and no whining.

In this chapter, we deal with the problem of vaginal inflammation—not a life-threatening problem, but still quite aggravating for those who suffer from it.

Vaginitis (the actual medical term) has both infectious and noninfectious causes. Most men are familiar with yeast infections, and may have heard of "trich" and bacterial vaginosis. Fewer men are aware of the common irritants that can cause significant vaginal and vulvar inflammation. In this chapter we will cover the symptoms, diagnosis, and treatments for each of the major causes of vaginitis.

Can men get vaginitis? Not unless they have a vagina (and that's an entirely different conversation). However, anything that causes vaginitis in a woman can cause irritation and inflammation of her partner's genitals through sexual contact. Men can spread vaginitis from one woman to another if they have more than one sexual partner. Also, women with vaginitis aren't able to have intercourse. So in reality, men are also afflicted by vaginitis when their partners have it.

By reading Chapter 3, you'll learn how to be a Supportive Guy if your partner has vaginitis.

GUY-Q TEST

1. Yeast infections are more common in women:
   a. taking certain antibiotics to treat an infection.
   b. having sex with someone else who has a yeast infection.
   c. who douche too often.
   d. all of the above.

2. Frequent recurrences of yeast may be prevented by:
   a. finishing the entire course of medication once begun.
   b. losing excess weight.
   c. avoiding the use of irritating chemicals in the vaginal area.
   d. wearing loose-fitting clothing.
   e. all of the above.

3. Bacterial vaginosis and trichomoniasis:
   a. are *not* carried by sexual partners.
   b. cause vaginal irritation and discharge.
   c. can be treated only with oral antibiotics.

4. The organism that causes a Trichomonas infection is:
   a. a bacteria.
   b. a virus.
   c. a protozoan.

5. Bacterial vaginosis in pregnancy may cause:
   a. an odorous discharge from the vagina.
   b. an increased risk of premature labor.
   c. an increased risk of uterine infection after delivery.
   d. all of the above.

6. Common items that may irritate the vagina include:
   a. deodorant soaps.
   b. fragrant douches.

c. tampons or other objects left in the vagina.

d. perfumed or colored toilet paper.

e. all of the above.

7. Atrophic vaginitis occurs when:

   a. a woman goes without estrogen for a prolonged period
   of time.

   b. a tampon is left in the vagina for too long.

   c. the vagina becomes infected and resists treatment.

8. If your partner has vaginitis, you could help by:

   a. encouraging her to consult with her doctor.

   b. being checked by your doctor if you have symptoms of
   genital irritation.

   c. not having intercourse with her until she's fully recovered.

   d. all of the above.

9. Men can become infected with:

   a. yeast.

   b. trichomoniasis.

   c. bacterial vaginosis.

   d. all of the above.

10. Your girlfriend is worried that she will catch a vaginal infection from your toilet seat; you should:

    a. reassure her that toilet seats usually are not contagious.

    b. take the hint and clean your whole apartment, especially the toilet seat.

    c. a and b.

Key: 1. d   2. e   3. b   4. c   5. d   6. e   7. a   8. d   9. d   10. c

YEAST INFECTIONS

Yeast is a fungus that is often a normal inhabitant of the vagina. It has been found in up to 70% of healthy women.

The vagina is not a sterile environment: it plays host to a multitude of microorganisms. In the normal state, these tiny life-forms do not disturb their host. When the balance between the different organisms is disrupted, however, one overgrows the others and causes problems. This is precisely the case with yeast infections.

Roughly 80% of yeast infections are caused by Candida albicans; the remaining 20% are caused by other Candida species, such as glabrata and tropicalis. This is important because the less common species are more likely to resist common drug treatments.

What Symptoms Do Yeast Infections Cause?

When yeast overgrows, it causes itching, redness, and a thick white discharge in most women. It can occur inside the vagina, on the vulva, or in both locations at once. Systemic (throughout the body) yeast infections also occur, but they are rare in healthy women. They are seen more often in people with compromised immune systems, like those with cancer or AIDS.

What Are the Risk Factors for Getting a Yeast Infection?

A yeast infection can happen at any time, but certain factors increase a woman's risk. These factors include taking antibiotics (for example, to treat a bladder infection), using high-dose birth control pills, having diabetes, or being pregnant. Women with depressed immunity, from a disease such as AIDS or because of certain medications (e.g., steroids), will likely have more yeast infections. Even wearing tight-fitting pants or shorts may increase a woman's chances of developing a yeast infection.

Yeast infections often occur in monogamous couples. Don't assume she has another partner if she has developed yeast; that often isn't true.

How Is Yeast Diagnosed?

The most common symptom of a yeast infection is genital itching; it can be quite intense. Many women also experience an increase in their discharge and burning with urination, caused by irritation of the vulva. They also may complain of pain during intercourse. Examination of the vagina and/or vulva often will show discharge and some degree of redness, swelling, and tenderness. There is an absence of "lumps, bumps, or craters," which might suggest warts, herpes, or other diagnoses. There is no odor from yeast.

To diagnose a yeast infection, the gynecologist will take a small sample of the thick, "curdy" discharge from the vagina or vulva and examine it under a microscope. About 80% of infected women will have yeast organisms visible on microscopic exam. A measurement of pH (acidity) of vaginal fluid also can be done to exclude other diagnoses. A woman with a yeast infection will usually have normal vaginal pH unless she also has other infections.

 It helps us make a diagnosis if no vaginal medications or douches are used for two days before the exam. This is because these chemicals obscure the signs of infection we're looking for.

How Is Yeast Treated?

Antifungal medications such as Monistat and GyneLotrimin (trade names), which can now be purchased without a prescription, are usually effective against uncomplicated yeast infections. Creams or suppositories work equally well when applied directly to the genital area. It's important to use the medication for the full treatment course (usually seven days) to avoid a relapse. In cases of extreme discomfort, a corticosteroid cream can be added. We instruct our patients to avoid intercourse until the treatment is completed.

These medications can be used without concern during pregnancy. A longer treatment course (ten days instead of seven) may be necessary if the woman is pregnant since pregnancy promotes the growth of yeast.

New single-dose yeast infection treatments with oral fluconazole are available by prescription. There is a small risk of liver damage with these medications, but they may be the preferred treatment under certain circumstances; consultation with a doctor should be obtained before use.

Other treatments include gentian violet (a very messy purple liquid) and oral ketoconazole. Cure rates are no higher with oral treatment, and drug toxicity (liver damage) is a small but real risk.

What If Yeast Infections Keep Coming Back?

Frequent recurrences of yeast are a fairly common problem—and a very exasperating one. Contributing factors may be:

- **Partial treatment** Women who do not use the medicine for the necessary number of days put themselves at risk for recurrence.

- **Frequent douching** Women increase their risk of yeast infections if they douche more than once a month.

- **Use of irritating chemicals in the vagina** Scented toilet paper, soaps, tampons, and vaginal sprays can "set up" yeast infections by irritating the genital area.

- **Clothing** Tight jeans, wet bathing suits, nylon underwear, and panty hose can contribute to yeast infections.

- **Excess weight** Yeast likes to grow in damp skin folds. Weight loss may help.

- **Antibiotic use** Antibiotics often eliminate some of the normal bacteria of the vagina, allowing yeast to overgrow. Women taking long-term antibiotics for any reason may therefore suffer chronic yeast infections.

- **Depressed immunity** Recurrent yeast may be the result of a major systemic illness such as AIDS (sometimes the yeast infections can lead to the AIDS diagnosis). Most women with recurrent yeast and decreased immunity, however, do not have AIDS. They may have a minor defect in their immune system that predisposes them to yeast.

- **Reinfection from a sexual partner** A man with oral or genital yeast can reinfect his partner after she's been treated.

- **Infection with a resistant strain of Candida** As mentioned, drug resistance is more common with certain species of Candida. A longer treatment course or use of a different antifungal may be needed. Cultures of the yeast may be helpful in deciding the best treatment in these unusual cases.

- **Diabetes** Women with diabetes are more likely to have recurrences.

How Can Yeast Recurrences Be Eliminated?

Controlling recurrences of yeast can be accomplished in most patients with the following:

- **General measures** Wear cotton underwear and loose-fitting clothes; reduce sweets and dairy products; improve control of diabetes.

- **Longer treatment courses** Use the treatment for ten or fourteen days instead of seven.

- **Suppressive doses of medication before the recurrences** Use the antifungal for three nights before a menstrual period (if that's when the yeast reoccurs) for six months.

- **Changing other medication use** Use lower-dose birth control pills or change to a different method of contraception; use an antifungal cream while taking antibiotics; stop taking systemic steroids (under your doctor's supervision).

- **Ketoconazole** This systemic antifungal may be worth the small risk of toxicity if all else fails.

- **Examination and treatment of a woman's sexual partners**

How Do I Know If I Have a Yeast Infection?

Yeast can be a subtle infection in men. You can check yourself by looking at your genitals under a bright light. Look for patches of skin that are slightly pink and itchy. If you are uncircumsized, make sure to check beneath the foreskin of your penis. Men do *not* have a discharge from their penis or burning with urination from yeast. Oral yeast (thrush) causes white-colored patches in the mouth. You are at risk if your partner has yeast, you use systemic steroids, you have diabetes, or you have depressed immunity. If you're not sure if you have yeast, see your doctor.

How Are Yeast Infections in Men Treated?

Men are treated with antifungal creams or oral medications in the same way their partners are. If you think you have a *mild* genital yeast infection, you can apply some of the same cream she uses to the infected area twice a day for seven days.

Make sure *you* complete the course of treatment. If you do not see any improvement after three days, call your doctor.

BACTERIAL VAGINOSIS

What Is Bacterial Vaginosis?

Bacterial vaginosis has gone by a lot of different names in the past: nonspecific vaginitis, haemophilis vaginitis, and coryne-bacterium vaginitis. For a while it was known as Gardnerella, after one scientist who studied the infection extensively, Dr. Herman Gardner.

Why have so many names been used for this vaginal infection? Because bacterial vaginosis is polymicrobial: it is caused by many different species of bacteria.

In the section on yeast infections, we told you that the vagina is not sterile. When all of the normal bacteria are suppressed, perhaps from taking an antibiotic, the yeast overgrows and causes symptoms. In the case of bacterial vaginosis, certain bacteria overgrow while other bacteria and yeast are suppressed. Organisms such as Gardenerella vaginalis multiply in great numbers and cause the characteristic symptoms associated with this infection.

During this infection, the total concentration of bacteria in the vagina increases 100-fold!

Again, as in yeast infections, the mere presence of the offending organisms doesn't mean the woman has an infection. Up to half of uninfected women studied have *some* of the offending bacteria in their vaginal secretions. Symptoms are produced only when the organisms multiply to numbers far greater than normal. This infection can occur in women of all ages, during pregnancy, and even after hysterectomy.

What Symptoms Does Bacterial Vaginosis Cause?

The most common symptom of women with bacterial vaginosis is a discharge with a fishy odor. This is found most often during and after a period or after intercourse. Mild burning or itching in the genital area may be present as well.

How Is Bacterial Vaginosis Diagnosed?

The diagnosis of bacterial vaginosis begins by noting a woman's symptoms. She will usually complain of an increase in vaginal discharge with odor and some burning or irritation in the genital area. Other symptoms, such as fevers, pelvic pain, or the presence of sores in the genital area might suggest other diagnoses. We also inquire whether she has had similar complaints in the past, and what their cause was.

Confirmation of the diagnosis is made during the pelvic exam, when a small amount of the discharge is obtained for evaluation. The bacteria can be seen under the microscope, attached to vaginal cells that were shed ("clue cells"). The pH (acidity) of the vaginal fluid is often altered because of the suppression of normal acid-producing bacteria. Finally, a "whiff" test is performed: a few drops of potassium hydroxide are added to the discharge sample, and a strong fishy odor is noted.

It is possible for bacterial vaginosis to occur along with yeast or other infections. During the pelvic exam, therefore, the gynecologist will attempt to exclude the presence of any other causes of infection or inflammation. Additional lab tests are done as indicated. Any suspicious lesions are examined and biopsied if necessary.

How Is Bacterial Vaginosis Treated?

Treatment of routine bacterial vaginosis is usually simple. The best antibiotics to suppress the overgrown populations of bacteria are metronidazole or clindamycin. Metronidazole is more widely used; it is given twice a day for seven days, and has a 95% cure rate. A single (larger) oral dose is almost as effective (85%) and may be the best choice for some patients. A metronidazole vaginal gel is also available; it should be used twice a day for five days. Patients taking metronidazole cannot drink *any* alcohol. This antibiotic is related to disulfiram, a medicine taken by alcoholics to remain sober; any ingestion of alcohol causes severe nausea and vomiting. Metronidazole is otherwise a very safe drug.

Clindamycin is taken twice a day orally for seven days, with a cure rate of greater than 90%. A two-percent clindamycin cream is just as effective when used once daily in the vagina for seven days.

As with other types of vaginitis, gynecologists recommend "pelvic rest" (translation: no intercourse) until the infection has resolved.

Is This an Important Infection in Pregnant Women?

Treatment of bacterial vaginosis in pregnancy is crucial. Current research suggests an increased risk of premature birth as well as infection inside the uterus during or after delivery. Clindamycin can be used at any time during pregnancy.

Metronidazole is not used during the first three months of pregnancy because of concerns over birth defects (probably unfounded), but it can be used later. Because of the potential risks from infection, women are treated in pregnancy whether or not they have symptoms.

Nonpregnant women with bacterial vaginosis but no symptoms often are not treated. An important exception is if surgery is planned: studies show a higher rate of infection after gynecologic surgery if these bacteria are present.

How Are Recurrent Episodes of Bacterial Vaginosis Treated?

Recurrent infections of bacterial vaginosis are common. The following steps may help reduce the frequency of repeat episodes:

- repeating the antibiotic treatment, either with the same drug or with another antibiotic that the bacteria are more sensitive to;

- using careful personal hygiene: wiping from "front to back" after using the toilet keeps bacteria from being dragged from the rectum into the vagina;

- treatment of sexual partners: some physicians will treat partners of women with recurrent infections even if they have no symptoms;

- use of dilute hydrogen peroxide douche to decrease odor;

- use of condoms if semen seems to aggravate her condition;

- povidone-iodine vaginal pessaries: when used for two weeks, these may be helpful.

How Do I Know If I Have Bacterial Vaginosis?

Men with this infection will typically have mild symptoms; burning with urination or a slight discharge from the head of their penis. A partner with recurrent episodes of this infection should prompt a responsible male to check for these signs and see a physician.

How Is This Infection in Men Treated?

Use of the same oral antibiotics used for women with bacterial vaginosis is effective in men. Make sure that you finish the full course of medicine if you are diagnosed with bacterial vaginosis.

TRICHOMONIASIS

The third entry in the infectious vaginitis category is tri-chomoniasias ("trich"). Caused by a protozoan organism known as Trichomonas vaginalis, this infection makes up 5–10% of vaginal infections.

Trichomonas differs from yeast infections and bacterial vaginosis in that it is usually acquired during intercourse. Very rarely it has been found in women who have never had sex. This suggests that it also can be acquired from an infected surface. It might really be true that a woman could become infected after contact with a contaminated toilet seat.

What Symptoms Does Trich Cause?

Women with trichomoniasis (infection with Trichomonas) usually complain of a sudden increase in vaginal discharge and genital irritation. A Trichomonas infection might also go unnoticed.

How Is Trich Diagnosed?

A pelvic examination will reveal an odorous, frothy green discharge along with redness and swelling of the genital tissues. Microscopic inspection of the vaginal discharge shows the organisms "swimming" (they propel themselves by moving their tails) and an increase in white blood cells. As in bacterial vaginosis, the acidity (pH) is altered because of the suppression of normal acid-producing bacteria.

Other means of diagnosis are less commonly used. Culture for the organism is not widely available, and Pap smears are likely to be inaccurate. A monoclonal antibody (blood) test is under development. It should help in the diagnosis of difficult cases.

As mentioned earlier in this chapter, during the examination the gynecologist will look for any other infections or abnormalities that also may be present.

How Is Trich Treated?

Treatment of this infection is usually a simple affair. Trich is very sensitive to the antibiotic metronidazole, which can be given orally in a single large dose or in smaller doses over five to seven days. See the previous section on bacterial vaginosis for more information on this drug.

Pregnant women receive the same treatment unless they acquire the infection during the first trimester of pregnancy (the first twelve weeks, when the organs of the baby are forming); during this time, clotrimazole cream can be used. It is important to eradicate this infection during pregnancy, since it has been associated with premature delivery and post-cesarean infections.

How Are Recurrent or Resistant Infections Treated?

Resistant infections (those still present after a complete course of antibiotics) are treated as follows:

- repeating the course of antibiotics;
- culturing the organism and testing for antibiotic sensitivity—then re-treating with an antibiotic the Trichomonas is more sensitive to;
- treating the sexual partner(s) to avoid reinfection;
- using vaginal treatment with metronidazole gel;
- using intravenous metronidazole: on rare occasions, high-dose intravenous antibiotics are needed.

How Do I Know If I Have Trichomoniasis?

Symptoms in men include burning with urination or a slight amount of discharge at the head of the penis. It is also possible to be infected and have no symptoms.

Since this is a sexually transmitted infection, sexual partners are usually treated as well.

How Is Trichomoniasis in Men Treated?

The same oral antibiotics used by women are effective for men with this infection. It is crucial to finish the full course of treatment once you start, even if the symptoms resolve quickly.

NONINFECTIOUS VAGINITIS: COMMON IRRITANTS

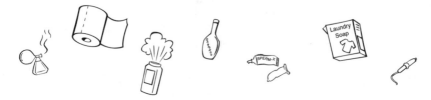

Is Vaginitis Always the Result of an Infection?

Irritation of the vagina and/or vulva from noninfectious causes is more common than most people appreciate. Genital tissues owe their exquisite sensitivity to thin skin and an abundance of nerves. It is this same anatomic makeup that causes the vagina and vulva to be so sensitive to irritation and injury. Thankfully, most cases of noninfectious vaginitis heal rapidly and completely once the offending agent is removed.

What Kinds of Complaints Do These Irritants Cause?

Symptoms of this type of vaginitis may be difficult to differentiate from symptoms caused by infections, such as yeast, Trichomonas, or bacterial vaginosis. Women will often complain of an increase in their discharge with an accompanying odor. In addition, they often notice vaginal and/or vulvar itching and/or discomfort.

How Is Noninfectious Vaginitis Diagnosed?

The diagnosis begins by obtaining a thorough history of a woman's complaints. The pelvic examination will reveal redness and swelling in the genital area. Microscopic examination of her discharge will show an increase in white blood cells (the body's primary defense against infection or irritation). The gynecologist also will look for the *absence* of an infection or other skin lesions. Sometimes a retained tampon or other "foreign body" is found in the vagina and the mystery is easily resolved.

How Is This Form of Vaginitis Treated?

Treatment of noninfectious vaginitis is usually simple. Removing the source of irritation is often all that's needed. Women suffering from significant discomfort can use a topical steroid cream in the genital area.

What Are the Types of Noninfectious Vaginitis?

The main causes of noninfectious vaginitis fall into three categories: chemical, physical, and atrophic vaginitis.

Chemical Vaginitis

The list of potential chemical irritants is limitless, but some of the more common causes are listed here:

- feminine deodorant sprays
- perfumed or colored toilet paper
- bubble bath or bath oils
- deodorant soaps
- laundry detergent (cold water formula) or fabric softeners with enzymes
- hot tubs or pools
- spermicides and/or condoms (latex allergy)
- disposable fragrant douches
- hair conditioners, dyes, or shampoos
- perfumes
- talcum powder
- over-the-counter medications

Physical or Foreign-Body Vaginitis

Physical or foreign-body vaginitis can be caused by the following:

- sanitary napkins with plastic shields
- condoms or diaphragms
- exercise bicycles
- horseback riding

- rowing machines
- tampons
- frequent use of small sanitary pads
- synthetic underwear (noncotton)
- tampons or other objects left in the vagina
- sex toys (vibrators, etc.)
- frequent masturbation
- pessaries

Atrophic Vaginitis

Women who have experienced menopause have skin changes in the genital area. Since the tissues there depend on estrogen, the decline in estrogen during menopause causes the tissues to become thinner, or "atrophic."

This weakening of the skin in the vagina and vulva can increase the risk of infection. In addition, the atrophic vagina can produce irritative symptoms on its own.

Symptoms of atrophic vaginitis are dryness, discomfort with intercourse, and a watery yellow discharge. In an estrogen-deficient (typically postmenopausal) woman, the diagnosis is made by excluding other causes of vaginitis by history and examination. The discharge contains an increase in white blood cells when viewed under the microscope.

Treatment of atrophic vaginitis consists of estrogen replacement. Vaginal estrogen creams provide more rapid relief than oral estrogen. Often oral and vaginal estrogen are used together. Relief from the irritative symptoms may take a few weeks to months of consistent treatment.

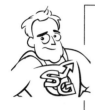

If Your Partner Has Vaginitis:

Now's the time to show her you're a Supportive Guy! Although vaginitis isn't a life-threatening problem, she will surely appreciate the following:

- Be patient. She may not be able to have intercourse for a few days or weeks. Even with the right treatment, the inflammation can be slow to resolve. Ask her how she's feeling, both physically and emotionally, about her problem.

- Encourage visits to the doctor. If she has significant vaginal complaints that are not resolving, she may have a more serious problem.

- Encourage compliance with treatment. If she has been prescribed a medication, help her remember to use it for the full course. If she has a problem with her medication, urge her to tell her doctor and not just stop using it.

- Don't add to the problem. If you use any chemicals on your genitals, make sure your partner knows about it. Be alert to the possibility it could be causing her problems.

POST TEST

1. Penicillin is the treatment of choice for yeast infections.
   T or F

2. Pregnancy increases the chances of developing a yeast infection.
   T or F

3. Yeast often can be successfully treated with over-the-counter antifungal creams.
   T or F

4. Bacterial vaginosis may cause a discharge with a fishy odor.
   T or F

5. The treatment of bacterial vaginosis is very important in pregnant women, even if they have no symptoms.
   T or F

6. Metronidazole is an effective antibiotic for both trich and bacterial vaginosis.
   T or F

7. Treatment of sexual partners is unnecessary if trichomoniasis is found.
   T or F

8. Men with Trichomonas infection will have no symptoms.
   T or F

9. Lower estrogen levels associated with menopause may lead to complaints of vaginal irritation.
   T or F

10. A number of physical and chemical agents that come into contact with the vaginal area may cause complaints similar to infectious vaginitis.
    T or F

Key: 1. F   2. T   3. T   4. T   5. T   6. T   7. F   8. F   9. T   10. T

BUMPS, DRIPS, AND OWIES

4

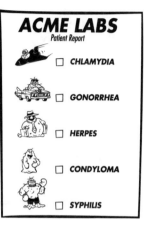

"Good afternoon, Jerry. What brings you here today?"

"Well, uh . . ."

"I'm sorry, Jerry. I didn't catch that."

"Um, Doc, I . . ."

"Yes . . . ? Are you having a problem?"

"No . . . It's just that I . . . There's this thing, *you see . . ."*

"Oh. Where is this—"

"On my, you know . . . my . . . THING!"

"Your penis?"

"Yeah!"

"Well, let's have a look!"

(Long pause.)

"Um, Doc, I gotta go now . . ."

Sexually transmitted diseases, or STDs as they're called in our practice, are not a new problem. Stories of various infections passed from person to person while engaged in various forms of lovemaking are as old as antiquity, and owing to the endless popularity of the "pleasures of the flesh," they will probably always be around.

It is not the intention of this chapter to debate any moral or religious questions that the practice of sex, whether in the bounds of marriage or, as it occasionally occurs, outside of said institution, may invite; rather, we intend to act here as we do in the office: as coaches and occasionally as referees in the Big Game of Love. From time to time, and sometimes too often, we are forced to throw the flag, stop the game, and issue a penalty. Usually it's a minor infraction with no significant losses; unfortunately, sometimes the whole game is lost.

What we're saying with this androgynous analogy is that STDs can have *serious* consequences. Chlamydia and gonorrhea can cause chronic pain and infertility, the virus that causes venereal warts can cause cervical cancer, herpes is a lifelong gift that most would like to return, and syphilis can make you lose both bladder control and your mind. All this without mentioning the disease most of you would have thought of first: AIDS, which, because of its well-known consequences, has finally turned the lights on for many people.

But the statistics that we follow as physicians lead us to believe that people aren't getting the message about STDs.

Chlamydia and gonorrhea are still very popular. Herpes infects millions, and syphilis is fighting to regain its old notoriety. There is literally an epidemic of venereal wart virus transmission. Worst of all, HIV infection is growing steadily in the heterosexual community (see Chapter 5).

When you read this chapter, we think you'll be impressed with all *you* can do to keep from becoming or begetting another statistic. At the very least, check out the section on the proper use of condoms. Admittedly, condoms are an ancient and unexciting method of disease and pregnancy prevention, but they are pretty effective when used correctly. Some improvements in technology are not unlikely, and soon we may even see condoms equipped with airbags for the safety conscious.

After many years in practice, we are too realistic to expect that your male urges will disappear. With this chapter, we hope merely to enlighten you with useful information on the most common sexually transmitted diseases: chlamydia, gonorrhea, venereal warts, herpes, and syphilis. Then, let your conscience and your knowledge be your guide.

Common sense says that you should know something about STDs as well as contraception (see Chapter 2) if you have a sexual relationship with a woman. Many men seem to know very little about either. Reading the information provided here will improve the chances that neither of you will ever regret the intimacy you share.

GUY-Q TEST

1. Chlamydia is:
   a. *not* a flower.
   b. a sexually acquired infection.
   c. an important cause of tubal blockage and infertility.
   d. all of the above.

2. Treatment for chlamydia includes:
   a. taking antibiotics.
   b. testing and treating sexual partners.
   c. both a and b.

3. Gonorrhea is different from chlamydia in that:
   a. it usually causes more symptoms.
   b. it usually causes fewer symptoms.
   c. there is no effective treatment.
   d. it can be passed from person to person by a handshake.

4. Women with gonorrhea may complain of:
   a. severe pelvic pain, fevers, and discharge.
   b. only mild discomfort in the pelvic area or no symptoms at all.
   c. either a or b.

5. Condyloma, or venereal warts, are:
   a. acquired by exposure to Chlamydia trachomatis.
   b. acquired by having sexual contact with someone with the Human Papilloma Virus.
   c. extremely contagious.
   d. b and c.

6. The venereal wart virus can infect:
   a. the cervix.
   b. the vagina.
   c. the skin outside the vagina.
   d. all of the above.

7. Herpes is:
   a. a viral infection.
   b. a lifelong infection.
   c. acquired by sexual contact.
   d. all of the above.

8. Strategies to prevent genital herpes recurrences include:
   a. acyclovir, an antiviral drug.
   b. antifungal creams.
   c. reducing physical and emotional stress.
   d. a and c only.

9. Signs of a syphilis infection may include:
   a. a painless ulcer in the genital area.
   b. fevers, lymph gland enlargement, and mouth ulcers.
   c. periods of time with no symptoms despite active disease.
   d. headaches, seizures, and memory loss.
   e. all of the above.

10. Protection from sexually transmitted diseases:
    a. is not an important concern for today's man.
    b. is only important if today's man wants to be around tomorrow.

Key: 1. d   2. c   3. a   4. c   5. d   6. d   7. d   8. d   9. e   10. b

CHLAMYDIA

What Is Chlamydia?

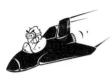

Chlamydia is not some kind of herbal tea. It is one of the most commonly diagnosed STDs and a major risk to female fertility; it prevents many couples from ever conceiving a child. Caused by a tiny, fragile bacteria (Chlamydia trachomatis) that can only survive within host cells, this infection has amazing stealth characteristics: *it often causes no symptoms in those exposed.* A woman with this infection rarely feels sick enough to visit the doctor, but may simply note a slight increase in her vaginal discharge, burning with urination, or mild pelvic pain. Her gynecologist usually will be unable to tell *when* she became infected, despite sophisticated diagnostic tests.

Chlamydia has been found in three percent of women tested on routine examination and in about one in five women attending STD clinics.* Women at particularly high risk are those 15 to 29 years old, unmarried, poor, members of a racial minority, and with multiple sexual partners. However, all sexually active women are at risk.

How Is Chlamydia Diagnosed?

The diagnosis of this subtle bug is usually made by performing a lab test on a swab of fluid from the cervix—an Enzyme Immuno-Assay (EIA). Results are close to 100% accurate and can be confirmed by a cell culture when necessary.

A gynecologist might be suspicious and obtain a chlamydia (EIA) test in the following circumstances:

- vague, mild pelvic pain in a sexually active woman;
- on examination, the cervix appears irritated, with a purulent (pus-filled) discharge.

It's also important to note that many women—or men—who think they have had chlamydia in the past may be mistaken. This false diagnosis occurs because doctors sometimes begin treating people for chlamydia before test results come back.

*W. E. Stamm and K. K. Holmes, "Chlamydia trachomatis infections of the adult" in K. K. Holmes et al., *Sexually transmitted diseases*, 2nd ed. New York: McGraw Hill, 1990, pp. 181–193.

Gynecologists and our primary-care colleagues have long made it a priority not to miss the opportunity to treat chlamydia because of its potential to harm the reproductive tract. Therefore, at times a doctor will treat someone for chlamydia at the same time he or she sends the tests to the lab (before the diagnosis is certain).

The well-meaning physician might tell the patient, "I think it's possible you have a chlamydia infection, and so I want to treat you now to make sure we get rid of it right away." By the time the woman gets home, she's upset enough to tell her partner, "the doctor thinks I have chlamydia!" which is only a short jump to believing she actually does. Occasionally the test comes back negative but she never finds out. The implications of a false diagnosis of pelvic infection are discussed later in this chapter.

One circumstance that *correctly* prompts treatment for chlamydia before test results are known is if a patient is diagnosed with gonorrhea. Studies have shown that gonorrhea and chlamydia infections often occur together, so when treating gonorrhea, gynecologists typically prescribe addi-tional antibiotics to cover chlamydia.

How Is Chlamydia Treated?

Once the chlamydia diagnosis is made by a reliable test, treatment consists of an oral antibiotic: tetracycline, doxycycline, azithromycin or, if the patient is pregnant, erythromycin. Other antibiotics are used less commonly. Sexual partners should be tested and treated with the same antibiotics. The antibiotics are routinely effective, with cure rates greater than 95%.

What If It's Not Treated?

Why all this concern over such a painless disease? Simply stated, while an infected woman may feel well, this stealthy bug could be destroying her fallopian tubes, a condition known as chlamydia salpingitis.

If you're wondering if chlamydia salpingitis is a significant cause of infertility, one study of infertile women with blocked tubes found that 50% had no knowledge of prior pelvic infection (i.e., they probably had chlamydia in the past).

D. E. Moore et al., "Increased frequency of serum antibodies to chlamydia trachomatis in infertility due to tubal disease," *Lancet* 2: 579 (1982); and D. W. Gump, S. Dickstein, and M. Gibson, "Endometritis related to chlamydia trachomatis infections," *Annals of Internal Medicine* 95: 61 (1981).

How Do I Know If I Have Chlamydia?

If you have chlamydia, you might experience some burning with urination or notice a slight discharge (milky, yellow fluid) on your underwear when you take them off. Or you may have no symptoms but you've been exposed to someone who has chlamydia. This infection has been called nonspecific urethritis (NSU) in the past.

How Do I Keep from Getting It?

Condoms work well in preventing chlamydia *if used correctly* (i.e., removed from the package and actually placed on the penis for the duration of intercourse).

If you think you might be infected, get tested. If you have chlamydia, get treatment and have your partner treated also.

GONORRHEA

What Is Gonorrhea?

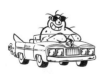

Gonorrhea (Neisseria gonorrhea) is the Cadillac of STDs. No stripped-down infection, it comes with loads of symptoms: pelvic pain, fevers, vaginal bleeding and/or discharge, burning with urination, and more. Where chlamydia is often subtle and quiet, gonorrhea plays like a rock band in your neighbor's garage: it's pretty hard to miss. Although it is possible to have only mild symptoms (if the infection resides solely within the cervix), it is not uncommon for people to be so ill they require hospitalization for intravenous antibiotics, fluids, and pain medications (see "What if it's not treated," below).

The typical incubation period from time of exposure until symptoms develop is two to seven days. The most common time in the menstrual cycle for a woman to develop symptoms is just after her menstrual period, when the flow of blood through the cervix allows easy passage for the bacteria into the upper genital tract (uterus, tubes, and ovaries). All sexually active people are at risk for this infection, but like chlamydia it is more common in young, unmarried, poor women with multiple sexual partners.

Far from being eradicated, gonorrhea grew steadily in the 70s and 80s; it is currently estimated (most cases are not reported) that close to two million cases of this infection occur in the United States each year.

How Is Gonorrhea Diagnosed?

Any sexually active woman coming to a doctor with pelvic pain, fevers, or an unusual discharge will likely be tested for gonorrhea. A rapid diagnosis can often be made with relative certainty in women through a microscopic exam of the cervical discharge: the tiny round gonococcus bacteria usually can be seen. Culture of the same cervical fluid takes longer (about three days) but provides more certainty. Usually these tests are run at the same time, and the decision to treat before the culture results are available may be made if the diagnosis seems likely. As is the case with chlamydia infection, untreated infection can be disastrous.

How Is Gonorrhea Treated?

A few oral and intravenous antibiotics are quite effective in ridding the body of this infection. The choice of drug and the duration of treatment are based on individual factors with each patient.

Patients are typically prescribed antibiotics to treat chlamydia at the same time they receive treatment for gonorrhea, because these two infections often occur together. Sexual partners should be tested and may be treated as well.

What If It's Not Treated?

Spread of this infection to the upper genital tract has both immediate and long-term consequences. Women can become acutely ill with severe pelvic pain, fevers, and marked fatigue; they may develop a pelvic abscess, joint involvement, or liver inflammation. When the infection is severe, a woman is said to have pelvic inflammatory disease. PID can be life-threatening and requires intravenous antibiotics to eradicate. Rarely, a woman requires major surgery to remove some or all of the infected pelvic organs. This kind of operation on a patient with a severe infection is one of the most challenging for a gynecologist.

Pregnant women with gonorrhea have an increased risk of miscarriage, premature delivery, arthritis, and systemic infection. Diagnosis and treatment is vital for mother and baby.

Long-term complications after an episode of PID could be pelvic pain and/or infertility caused by the damage left behind by the infection. One episode of PID leaves approximately 11% of women sterile; repeat infections raise this number significantly. Like chlamydia, gonorrhea can scar and ruin fallopian tubes. It can bind the ovaries to the intestines or the uterus, causing pain with exercise or intercourse. Both chronic pain and infertility are problems of enormous magnitude, both physically and emotionally, for our patients.

How Do I Know If I Have Gonorrhea?

Gonorrhea historically was called the Clap, from the French "clapois," referring to the swollen lymph nodes that occur with severe infection. Men usually notice burning and/or frequency of urination and a purulent (pus-filled) penile discharge. If ignored in the male, the infection can cause sterility by destroying the testicles.

If you think you might be infected, get tested. If you have gonorrhea, get treatment and make sure your partner does also.

How Do I Keep from Getting It?

Condoms prevent infection with Neisseria gonorrhea in almost all instances, when used properly. If you're unsure about your partner's health status, abstinence is the best option.

CONDYLOMA

What Is Condyloma?

Condyloma, or infection with Human Papilloma Virus (HPV), has been the most common STD seen in our OB/GYN offices for several years. This virus causes only mild symptoms and is extremely contagious.

Estimates of the prevalence of HPV in the lower genital tract among "healthy" women (those with no complaints or obvious signs of infection) range from 9 to 29%. These statistics represent an *enormous* number of people, both male and female, whose lives are being adversely affected.

One recent study showed that 46% of nearly 500 women visiting a university health service for various complaints had DNA evidence of exposure to HPV.

H. Bauer et al., "Genital human papilloma virus infection in women university students as determined by PCR-based method," *Journal of the American Medical Association* 265: 472 (1991).

The most common forms of condyloma are venereal warts and flat condyloma. You may be familiar with venereal warts, little cauliflower-like eruptions that occur on the penis, scrotum, vagina, and vulva. Flat condyloma are raised, plateau-like lesions that can be found on the cervix and vulva.

When the infection involves the cervix, it can also cause dysplasia, or precancerous changes. Of the more than 60 subtypes of the virus, only a few are capable of this behavior; the majority merely cause infection of the cervix, so-called koilocytotic changes. Rarely, infection with a particularly nasty subtype of the virus can cause rapid progression of dysplasia to true cervical cancer, so we follow all infected patients closely until their Pap smears revert to normal (see Chapter 7).

How Long Does It Take from Exposure to the Virus Until It Causes Warts to Appear?

The time from exposure until expression of the infection, or the "incubation time," is between three weeks and eight months, with an average of just under three months. The virus can be in a latent, or inactive, state for a prolonged period of time; we don't know yet how long that may be, but experience suggests it may be *years*. This means that the *same* infection may cause several lesions in the genital area over time as the virus becomes active in different areas.

We don't know all that we'd like to about condyloma, an uncomfortable admission, to be sure. Given our propensity in the medical profession for dispensing knowing glances and chin-holding *hmmms*, we are unfortunately left with our intellectual pants down when asked simple questions like, "When did I get this?" and "When will it be gone?" Alas, from the common cold to HPV to HIV, viruses continue to elude our complete understanding.

How Is Condyloma Diagnosed?

The typical female patient with HPV arrives in the office with venereal warts and/or an abnormal Pap smear. Biopsies (small tissue samples) may be taken of suspicious lesions on the cervix, the vulva, or the vagina for confirmation, but visual inspection and a history of sexual contact is usually enough.

How Is Condyloma Treated?

When the patient has venereal warts or flat condyloma, treatment is accomplished by applying chemicals like bi- or tri-chloro acetic acid (BCA or TCA) or podophyllin resin to the area. Several applications over a few weeks are often necessary. One prescription drug allows patients to self-treat on consecutive days at home, which may be more effective.

Recurrences in the same or nearby areas are not uncommon and must be monitored by the patient. Larger lesions or those not responding to treatment may be removed surgically or with laser treatment.

Treatment for cervical infection with HPV is still controversial; some doctors do not recommend treatment, while others use either BCA topical solution or cryotherapy (freezing). When precancer is found along with the HPV, the treatment is usually freezing or surgically removing the part of the cervix that is involved. Careful follow-up for a prolonged period with Pap smears is necessary to detect recurrences.

New medicines that work by enhancing local immune response against the virus are currently being evaluated. These include an immune system stimulator called imiquimod (trade name Aldara). This cream, which can be self-applied, has a 72% success rate. Clearance of the warts occurs in 4 to 16 weeks, which is similar to other treatments. Side effects are mild, usually just a local skin reaction with some redness and irritation.

Another option for treatment may be coming from Europe: Accusite gel. This is a medicine containing 5-Fluorouracil and epinephrine that is injected into the affected skin weekly for up to six weeks. Unfortunately its cure rate and rate of recurrences aren't significantly better than what's currently available.

Research is also underway on a vaccine that will prevent cervical cancer by stopping HPV from entering cells.

What If It's Not Treated?

Twenty to sixty percent of patients with this infection will recover without treatment, thanks to the immune system. However, certain subtypes of the virus may lead to cervical cancer. A greater risk of cancers of the vulva, vagina, and rectum has also been found.

Research has shown that a woman with HPV on her Pap smear has a 15-fold higher risk of developing cervical cancer than the general population.

H. Mitchell, M. Drake, and G. Medley, "Prospective evaluation of risk of cervical cancer after cytological evidence of HPV," *Lancet* 2: 573 (1986).

In men, there seems to be a slightly increased risk of penile cancer with HPV infection. Since the virus is very infectious, lack of adequate treatment also commonly leads to infection of sexual partners.

How Do I Know If I Have Condyloma?

Men with condyloma will usually have painless, cauliflower-like warts in the genital area. The warts may be very small and inconspicuous, but this appearance does not correlate with their ability to infect and harm others.

There are no blood tests or cell cultures to diagnose this infection; it must be identified visually by a trained professional.

 If you've been exposed to condyloma (HPV), or have a partner who's been diagnosed with it, have a knowledge-able practitioner examine you. It's not enough to have a quick look yourself.

How Do I Keep from Getting It?

Where have we heard this before? Condoms are helpful at reducing the spread of this and many other STDs. It's important to remember, however, that condoms won't protect areas other than the penis from this infection. If you are with a new partner who has this infection, avoid all genital contact until she's been treated.

Unfortunately, due to the nature of this virus, you may still get the infection even after your partner has been treated. Watch out for signs of HPV infection in yourself, and make an appointment for an exam if they occur.

HERPES

What Is Herpes?

Herpes is a viral infection that never leaves. Like your weird uncle Harold, it retreats into a back bedroom of your body, the dorsal root ganglion (a nerve bundle near the spinal cord), and then reinvites itself into your life whenever it pleases. More accurately, the infection tends to recur at times of physical or mental stress.

The herpes virus is usually most potent when it first appears. Women generally complain of painful blisterlike sores in and around the vagina, the cervix, and/or the rectum; sometimes fevers and generalized weakness accompany them. On very rare occasions, an infected man or woman may develop a severe systemic/nervous system infection, meningoencephalitis, during the first outbreak. Subsequent visitations of the virus are far less severe, and some lucky folks never have any after the first outbreak. Usually, no scarring or physical evidence of the disease remains after healing takes place.

The average number of viral outbreaks per year is three to four, lasting a few days each; the remainder of the time, people with herpes feel completely well. They are only infectious immediately before and during an outbreak. Symptoms of itching or burning at the site typically precede an outbreak. These symptoms are called the prodrome.

On rare occasions, the virus can be transmitted to a sexual partner even when the infected person is without lesions or symptoms. This is estimated to be possible less than one percent of the time.

Although its popularity in the press has been eclipsed of late by HIV, herpes is still a common problem: approximately 45 million adolescent and adult Americans have been infected with genital herpes. Research shows that nearly 20% of the population shows evidence on blood testing of exposure to the herpes virus.*

---

*D. T. Fleming et al., "Herpes simplex virus type 2 in the U.S., 1976–1994," *New England Journal of Medicine* 337: 1105–1111 (1997).

Many people have genital herpes but are unaware. In one recent study of reproductive-age women, only 5 percent reported a history of herpes.* However, about 30 percent of women in the United States have been shown to have herpes on blood testing.**

---

*C. Prober et al., "The management of pregnancies complicated by genital infection with herpes simplex virus," *Clinics of Infectious Disease* 15: 1031–1038 (1992).
**D. T. Fleming et al., "Herpes simplex virus type 2 in the U.S., 1976–1994," *New England Journal of Medicine* 337: 1105–1111 (1997).

How Is Herpes Diagnosed?

Genital herpes (HSV-2) can be diagnosed by visual inspection alone in a woman with characteristic painful, blisterlike lesions in the genital area who's had recent sexual contact. Swollen nearby lymph nodes and other associated symptoms, when present, help to make the diagnosis. The time from exposure to the virus to onset of symptoms is one to seven days.

If the examining physician isn't certain, he or she may take a sample of fluid from an open blister or an infected cervix and order a herpes culture; results are ready in a few days. Blood tests are not helpful in everyday practice because presence of antibodies to an extremely common virus, HSV-1, or oral herpes (the "cold sore" virus), can't be differentiated from genital herpes. Some research centers, however, use highly specialized tests which can tell HSV-1 from HSV-2. Presence of the antibody to the cold sore virus may help prevent the acquisition of genital herpes.

If this isn't confusing enough, oral herpes (type 1) can cause genital lesions after oral-genital contact, and genital herpes (type 2) may also cause oral or eye lesions.

How Is Herpes Treated?

The good news is that we now have a medicine that shortens the duration of primary and recurrent outbreaks and speeds their healing. Acyclovir (trade name Zovirax) reduces the suffering of herpes patients by inhibiting the growth of the responsible virus. This medicine is well tolerated and seems to be harmless to the rest of the body.

Other pharmaceutical companies are racing to develop a better antiviral for herpes sufferers. New medications are being released that offer similar effectiveness with less frequent dosings.

Another important use of acyclovir has been found. Studies have shown that taking the medication in smaller doses every day can greatly reduce the number of outbreaks. This treatment (suppressive therapy) is usually reserved for the rare patient unfortunate enough to have recurrences every few weeks.

 Reducing physical and emotional stress is an effective nonpharmacologic way to reduce the frequency of herpes outbreaks.

What If It's Not Treated?

Unlike chlamydia or gonorrhea, herpes is not caused by a bacteria that can be eliminated with an antibiotic. The use of antivirals *does not eliminate the virus*, but *can* play an important role in shortening the active disease interval and diminishing the severity of the illness. Many other treatments have been suggested, both homeopathic and traditional, because of the tremendous interest in, and *fear* of, this infection.

What Is Herpes Really Like for Those Who Have It?

Before the age of AIDS, herpes was the most dreaded result of unprotected sexual contact—more dreaded than any other sexually transmitted infection, perhaps more dreaded than unwanted pregnancy. Support groups formed all over the country to help people "put their lives back together" after acquiring this virus. Relationships ended, many people stopped socializing, some became severely depressed. There were unfounded fears about cancer, infertility, and long-term health problems.

Let's add up the stats on herpes for the *typical* infected person:

- Initial outbreaks usually cause mild to moderate pain in the genital area and last three to seven days;

- Three to four recurrences will occur per year, lasting two to five days each. This adds up to six to twenty days per year. The person looks and feels completely well at other times;

- Infectiousness is essentially limited to those times of pro-drome and active disease, and can be diminished further with the aid of acyclovir and other treatments;

- The disease does not damage the upper genital tract (i.e., the uterus, tubes, and ovaries) unlike gonorrhea and chla-mydia;

- Aside from a *minimally* increased risk of miscarriage, there is no association with infertility. Pregnant patients with HSV are otherwise managed the same as uninfected women, except they are screened in labor for active infec-tion. If detected, a cesarean section is recommended to pro-tect the newborn;

- Herpes has not been proven to cause cancer of the cervix or any other part of the body in women; the same is true for men.

Why has there been such a stigma surrounding herpes infec-tion? In the past, there were unfounded fears about its effects on the body. Perhaps the negativity and shame also reflects society's views about sex outside of marriage.

When a person reveals that they have herpes, they admit not only to having sex but also to getting a disease. For some, this conjures up images of illicit affairs, one-night stands, or even group sex. These stereotypes have little to do with how most people acquire herpes or any other STD.

It will be a good sign for our society when people are free to discuss their sexual past in relationships without fear of being unfairly judged.

How Do I Know If I Have Herpes?

This infection *can* be quite subtle, causing few if any symptoms. Typical symptoms in men are the same as for women: clusters of one- to two-millimeter (a little larger than the head of a pin) "pimples," or blisters, in the genital area. These may open after a day or two and become shallow ulcers. The lesions are intensely itchy and sensitive to the touch.

During the initial outbreak, you may also notice swollen lymph nodes in the groin area and generalized symptoms like fatigue, muscle aches, and weakness. Recurrences are usually much milder, and are often heralded by prodromal symptoms such as burning, itching, or tingling in the groin or down the legs.

 Don't be so sure that was an ingrown hair last week! If any of this sounds at all familiar, see your doctor the next time it happens. The love you save may be your own.

How Do I Keep from Getting It?

If a woman knows she has this infection, she'll probably tell you before you begin a sexual relationship together (just as we know you would!).

The best way to keep from getting herpes from an infected partner is to avoid sex during her infectious times and to use condoms, although, as in the case of all STDs, there are no guarantees.

If she has frequent outbreaks (once a month or more), her physician may recommend she take suppressive doses of acyclovir for her sake as well as yours. However, even this is not 100% effective in preventing transmission of the infection.

Currently, the University of California at San Diego, Department of Dermatology, is participating in a multicenter international trial investigating a herpes vaccine. If successful, this could prevent uninfected partners from getting the infection by making them immune. Anyone without genital herpes would be a candidate for the vaccine, if it is successful.

SYPHILIS

What Is Syphilis?

 Syphilis is an STD that has been around for centuries. Although other infections have been getting more press of late, this old fighter is on the rise and showing signs he hasn't lost his stuff. So, woe to the poor soul who ignores this one: Syphilis can cause fatal heart disease and severe neurologic problems, including loss of coordination and psychosis, if left untreated.

Syphilis is caused by a microscopic, spiral-shaped organism called Treponema pallidum, a member of the family Spirochaetacea. It was not discovered as the cause of syphilis until 1905, although the infection had been a major health problem in Europe since the seventeenth century. It is believed that syphilis was introduced to Europe in 1493 by sailors returning from the New World with Christopher Columbus—a bounty neither anticipated nor appreciated by the Queen of Spain.

Of further historical interest: Because of a perceived connection between syphilis and prostitution, brothels were sharply curtailed throughout Europe in the seventeenth century. A typical ordinance, like one passed in Paris in 1635, sentenced prostitutes to flogging, having their heads shaved, and exile without trial.

Because of exhaustive public health efforts and the discovery of effective treatments, the number of reported cases per year of syphilis declined in the United States from 106,000 in 1947 to 25,500 by 1975. The practice of testing all marriage license applicants for this disease is an example of the effectiveness of public health policy; it can lower the risk of syphilis transmission between partners, as well as to an infant born of their union.

 New cases of syphilis are on the rise, with a 75% increase in reported cases between 1985 and 1990. These cases have been concentrated in the southeast states and Texas, where a large immigrant population with limited access to health care resides.

Centers for Disease Control and Prevention; www.cdc.gov/nchs.

What Symptoms Does Syphilis Cause?

Syphilis is acquired through sexual contact (intercourse). Two to six weeks after sex with an infected person, the characteristic lesions of syphilis occur: painless, shallow ulcers up to three centimeters in size. These "chancres" are extremely infectious. The lesions are found most often on the vulva, but are also known to occur on the cervix, in the vagina, or near the anus. Distant chancres have been found on the nipple or in the mouth. Swollen nearby lymph nodes are sometimes seen as well. The ulcers heal without scarring in a few weeks regardless of treatment; however, the consequences of untreated infection can be severe and are discussed below.

How Is Syphilis Diagnosed?

Suspicion of syphilis is raised whenever a woman comes to us complaining of painless ulcers, as described above. Contact with an infected person would be a cause for concern as well, especially if the patient could describe a chancre on herself or her partner, whether healed or not.

Examination of the fluid from a fresh lesion, using a special microscopic technique (Dark-Field Microscopy), can demonstrate the organism immediately. The most commonly used tests for the diagnosis of syphilis are blood tests; however, these tests are often negative until the chancre has been present for one to two weeks and may need to be repeated if done too early.

How Is Syphilis Treated?

Syphilis was studied in the first half of the seventeenth century by a German doctor named Paracelsus, who was among the first to view disease as something that was acquired from *outside* the body.

The prevailing opinion in the seventeenth century was that diseases were caused from within, by an imbalance of body humors. Therefore, treatments consisted largely of purging and bloodletting. Imagine having the dual misfortune of having neurosyphilis and *not* being Dr. Paracelsus's patient! You might well have been carried, screaming, into the doctor's office, only to be bled a couple of quarts for your treatment. Afterward, if you were strong enough, you could mutter your thanks and pay the doctor's bill in chickens or whatever. Of course, old Dr. Paracelsus wasn't much help, either, although he was on the right track; he tried to cure people by giving them sulfur or mercury. Remember this the next time you complain about modern-day medical care.

The first effective treatment for syphilis was Salvarsan, discovered in 1909 by the German bacteriologist Paul Ehrlich. That Salvarsan was actually made from arsenic (a deadly poison) was probably not advertised. In 1943, penicillin was discovered to be effective, and it continues to be the drug of choice for syphilis today. Tetracycline and erythromycin are alternates when issues of drug allergy come up.

What If It's Not Treated?

So far we have only alluded to what might happen if someone with an acute, or primary, case of syphilis isn't treated. What follows is a brief description of the subsequent stages of this disease, as was learned over the centuries before effective treatment became available.

Secondary syphilis occurs about six weeks after the primary chancre heals. Since the Spirochete is still alive and well, it begins to wreak havoc throughout the body. Fevers, general lymph gland enlargement, mouth ulcers, and wartlike, flat, painless genital lesions called condyloma lata may occur. A characteristic skin rash that involves the soles of the feet and palms of the hands is also typical of this stage. Hair loss, eye inflammation, and meningitis (inflammation of the lining of the brain) may be seen as well. Blood tests remain positive during this stage, and most folks recognize they aren't quite well and seek effective treatment.

Latent syphilis occurs in two-thirds of untreated patients with secondary syphilis. The organism continues to replicate, but despite ongoing inflammatory changes throughout the body, there are no outward signs of its presence. This stage may last undetected for 20 to 30 years.

Tertiary syphilis results in one-third of untreated patients and comes in three forms:

- **Cardiovascular** Roughly 10% of patients have substantial destruction of heart tissue and major blood vessels, such as the aorta;
- **Gummatous** Patients may experience widespread damage to skin, bone, liver, cartilage, and other organs;
- **Neurosyphilis** Neurosyphilis can occur 5 to 35 years after the initial infection and can cause headaches, seizures, memory loss, loss of coordination and bladder control, and psychosis.

Syphilis in pregnancy can cause miscarriage or stillbirths, although routine prenatal testing makes this quite rare these days. Babies born to infected mothers are said to have congenital syphilis. They can suffer birth defects, including a skin rash and bone disease.

How Do I Know If I Have Syphilis?

The symptoms as described for women are essentially the same for men: characteristic painless ulcers, most commonly in the genital area, with or without swollen lymph glands nearby. These findings or contact with an infected partner should alert you to seek appropriate testing.

 Any sore in the genital area, *painful or not*, deserves inspection by a qualified health professional. People will remain infected with syphilis long after the ulcers heal unless they receive treatment.

How Do I Keep from Getting It?

If you have suspicions that your partner either has this infection or has been exposed to it, you should avoid sex until she's been adequately tested and treated. Remember that the disease can be quite active after the healing of the primary chancre, during the latent phase, without outward signs or symptoms. Again, condoms are a guy's best friend because they offer substantial protection against this and other STDs, as well as against unwanted pregnancy.

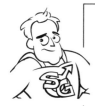

Using Condoms to Prevent HIV Infection and Other STDs

Latex condoms can greatly reduce a person's risk of acquiring or transmitting sexually transmitted diseases, including HIV infection. HIV is the virus that causes AIDS.

But for condoms to provide maximum protection, they must be used *consistently* and *correctly*.

Consistent use means using a condom from start to finish every time you have sex. Correct use means:

1. Use a new latex condom for each act of intercourse—whether vaginal, anal, or oral.

2. Be careful when opening the condom. Do not use your teeth, fingernails, or other sharp objects to open the condom wrapper—you might tear the condom inside.

3. Put the condom on after the penis is erect and before any sexual contact.

4. Hold the tip of the condom and unroll the condom all the way down the erect penis—the rolled rim should be on the outside. Leave space at the tip of the condom for semen, but make sure that no air is trapped in the condom's tip.

5. If additional lubrication is needed, lubricate the outside of the condom if it is not pre-lubricated. Use only water-based lubricants. You can purchase a lubricant at any pharmacy, and your pharmacist can tell you which lubricants are water-based. Oil-based lubricants, such as petroleum jelly, cold cream, hand lotion, cooking oil, or baby oil, weaken the condom.

6. Withdraw from your partner while the penis is still erect. Hold the condom firmly to keep it from slipping off.

7. Throw the used condom in the trash. Never reuse a condom.

8. If the condom breaks during sex, withdraw from your partner and put on a new condom.

(continued)

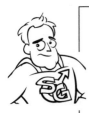

Always keep condoms handy, but store them in a cool, dry place that is out of direct sunlight. Do not use a condom after its expiration date or if it has been damaged in any way.

Latex condoms are available in different sizes, colors, and textures. Find the one that is right for you.

Novelty products are not effective in preventing STDs.

Not having sex is the best way to avoid getting HIV infection or other STDs. However, if you do have sex, condoms are highly effective in preventing STD transmission if used correctly from start to finish, each time you have intercourse.

Reprinted by permission from the Centers for Disease Control and Prevention, Office of HIV/AIDS. U.S. Department of Health and Human Services/Public Health Services.

POST TEST

1. Chlamydia infection in a woman often goes undetected.
   T or F

2. Nonspecific urethritis is the old name for chlamydia infection in men.
   T or F

3. Gonorrhea doesn't damage a woman's fallopian tubes.
   T or F

4. PID may be caused by a gonorrhea infection.
   T or F

5. Condyloma infection causes painful ulcers on the genital skin. These ulcers are difficult to ignore.
   T or F

6. The virus that causes venereal warts can often be found on the cervix.
   T or F

7. Herpes infections often cause infertility by scarring the tubes and ovaries.
   T or F

8. Herpes is the most common cause of abnormal Pap smears.
   T or F

9. Syphilis infections are increasingly common.
   T or F

10. Condoms are a man's best friend in new relationships.
    T or F

Key: 1. T   2. T   3. F   4. T   5. F   6. T   7. F   8. F   9. T   10. T

HIV/AIDS: WHAT YOU NEED TO KNOW, OR ELSE

5

AIDS The mere mention of the word causes pulses to quicken, palms to sweat. How many times have *you* wondered if you're infected with the AIDS virus?

Even if you've managed to stay HIV negative, AIDS has become a part of your life. Most of us know someone, or know someone who knows someone, who's died because of AIDS. Many of us know more than a few who are sick, or will someday soon become sick. Too sick to ever get well.

Lest we forget, the media assaults us daily with news about AIDS: famous people who have died from it, new drugs to be used in the fight against it, the ever-rising numbers of new AIDS cases. Day after day the epidemic rages on, no less frightening because we're used to hearing about it.

Why is AIDS so frightening? Because despite the media coverage, despite all the money being spent on research, despite the collective cry for help from around the world, the word *cure* is never mentioned. Those of us who have followed this disease since it first appeared know better than to hope for a cure right now. We listen instead for phrases like "prolonging the symptom-free interval" and "improving the quality of life." Although only temporary solutions, these treatments offer more than the relentless recountings of death we now must endure when we talk about this ravenous disease.

In the beginning, most of us were protected, we thought, from AIDS. Only those who were homosexual, received untested blood, or used intravenous drugs could get sick. The truth is far more scary because the AIDS boogeyman is actually under *everyone's* couch. The answer to "Who gets AIDS?" turns out to be *anyone*, particularly if they're sexually active.

If you are sexually active, you *must* learn about this disease. An ounce of prevention is worth a pound of cure, right? For the disease called AIDS, for the foreseeable future, that "ounce of prevention" could easily save your life.

GUY-Q TEST

1. AIDS is caused by:
   a. a bacteria.
   b. a virus.
   c. a protozoan.

2. Diagnosis of HIV infection is made by:
   a. a urine test.
   b. an ELISA blood test.
   c. the Eastern blot test.
   d. the ELISA and Western blot tests.

3. Symptoms of AIDS include:
   a. chronic diarrhea.
   b. unexplained fevers.
   c. memory loss.
   d. weight loss.
   e. all of the above.

4. Diseases associated with AIDS include:
   a. cervical cancer.
   b. Kaposi's sarcoma.
   c. Pneumocystis pneumonia.
   d. Tay-Sachs disease.
   e. all but d.

5. Zidovudine, an antiviral medication, may be used during pregnancy to:
   a. keep the mother from getting AIDS.
   b. help the fetus grow to a normal size.
   c. prevent premature delivery.
   d. lower the risk of the baby being HIV infected.

6. Those people at very high risk for HIV include:
   a. prostitutes.
   b. intravenous drug users.
   c. sexual partners of intravenous drug users.
   d. heterosexuals with multiple sex partners.
   e. all of the above.

7. Ways to prevent HIV infection include:
   a. openly discussing prior sexually transmitted diseases and HIV tests early in a relationship.
   b. practicing safe sex with one partner.
   c. not using intravenous drugs, or at least not sharing needles.
   d. taking daily antibiotics.
   e. all but d.

8. The practice of safe sex includes:
   a. abstaining from sexual intercourse.
   b. using a condom correctly each time.
   c. having sex with only one partner.
   d. all of the above.

9. Correct condom use means:
   a. latex condoms, not natural skin condoms.
   b. holding the end nearest your body upon withdrawal.
   c. use of condoms during oral sex also.
   d. all of the above.

Key: 1. b 2. d 3. e 4. e 5. d 6. e 7. e 8. d 9. d

HIV/AIDS

Why Do I Need to Know about HIV and AIDS?

The American Foundation for AIDS Research estimates that worldwide there are 33.4 million people infected with HIV, and the number is still increasing.

In the United States:

- More than 350,000 people are currently living with HIV or AIDS.

- The vast majority of women infected with HIV are between 15 and 45 years of age.

- Women accounted for more than one-third of reported cases of HIV infection as of June 1998.

- There were more than 5,000 new cases of HIV infection among women between July 1997 and June 1998.

- As of 1998, 39% of women acquired the infection from heterosexual contact. More than 38,000 women and 20,000 men have been infected this way.

- Between 1992 and 1997, an estimated 241,000 people in the United States died from AIDS; of these, more than 38,000 were women.

- AIDS is the number-one killer of Americans aged 25 to 44.

A fact:

- Although treatments for and survival rates from AIDS have markedly improved, there are no vaccines and no cures.

What Is AIDS?

Some definitions will help you understand this disease:

- **HIV** Human immunodeficiency virus, the virus that causes AIDS. It was discovered in Paris at the Pasteur Institute in 1983. A person who is infected with the virus is called HIV positive. Being HIV positive is different from having the *disease* known as AIDS.

- **Immunodeficiency** Disabling of the immune system. The HIV virus attacks a key element of this blood-borne system, the CD4 lymphocyte. As the numbers of these special lymphocytes decrease, the risk of developing AIDS increases.

- **Opportunistic infections** Infections that gain access only to people with weakened immunity. In other words, opportunistic infections "kick you while you're down." They are typical of AIDS because the disease takes such a toll on the immune system. Examples are toxoplasmosis, systemic fungal infections, and Pneumocystis pneumonia.

- **ARC** AIDS-Related Complex. Persons with ARC are not well, but not sick enough yet to qualify as having AIDS. They already have some degree of immunodeficiency. (The term *ARC* is no longer commonly used.)

- **AIDS** Acquired immunodeficiency syndrome, the disease that results from infection with the HIV virus. This virus attacks and disables the immune system, the body's primary defense against infection and disease.

Many different infections, diseases, and even cancers can develop in an AIDS patient. Common examples of AIDS-defining illnesses in people known to be HIV positive are Pneumocystis pneumonia and Kaposi's sarcoma (a skin cancer common in male AIDS patients). Cervical cancer has also been added as an AIDS-defining illness in women (if the woman is HIV positive).

How Is AIDS Diagnosed?

AIDS is diagnosed through a blood test. A small amount of blood is drawn and then tested for antibodies to the HIV virus. If this screening test is negative, the person either doesn't have the infection or has not yet produced antibodies to it. On rare occasions, the test may be falsely negative (less than one percent of tests).

If the initial test is positive, a second, confirmatory test is done on the blood sample before the result is released. This is because the screening test *very* rarely misidentifies someone as having the virus when they don't. Often, a positive test is repeated within two weeks as an additional confirmation.

The first test for HIV in most labs is called an Elisa, for Enzyme-Linked Immunosorbent Assay. Blood is tested by adding an enzyme that triggers a color change when the HIV antibody is detected in the blood. The Elisa correctly identifies someone as having the virus more than 99% of the time. The confirmatory test is called the Western blot, and it is also highly accurate. The Elisa test has been used to screen all donated blood for HIV in the United States since 1985.

The timing of HIV tests is crucial. If someone is tested too soon after becoming infected, the test will be negative. Because the tests look for antibodies to the virus and not for the virus itself, a person recently infected by the virus may have negative test results. It takes between six weeks and six months for antibodies to appear in an infected person's blood.

A new way to diagnose HIV infection without blood testing is currently being developed. Called Orasure, it uses a special cotton swab to rub the tissue between the gums and cheek. The fluid collected is tested for the AIDS virus. A blood test is still needed to confirm the results.

What Are the Symptoms of AIDS?

Being HIV positive is not the same as having the disease known as AIDS. Actually, most people infected with the HIV virus don't get sick for some time. Currently, only a small percentage of people acquiring the HIV virus develop AIDS in the first five years.

At the time of initial infection with the HIV virus, people often develop a flu-like illness. It typically occurs two to four weeks after exposure and includes fever, muscle aches, sore throat, headache, and swollen lymph nodes. Most infected individuals recover from this mild illness within two weeks and feel well for a number of years afterward.

AIDS occurs once the immune system has been disabled by the virus (HIV). Common symptoms are weight loss, fatigue, memory loss, chronic diarrhea, and night sweats. On physical examination, women may have recurrent vaginal yeast infections, precancer of the cervix, or swollen lymph nodes. Loss of vision, weakness or lack of coordination, and certain skin problems are often detectable in women or men with AIDS. However, the great majority of people who have these symptoms do not have HIV infection or AIDS.

As the disease progresses, opportunistic infections such as Pneumocystis pneumonia, toxoplasmosis, cytomegalovirus infection, and tuberculosis may occur. Neurologic symptoms, as mentioned above, including dementia and psychosis, are seen. Certain cancers, including Kaposi's sarcoma, leukemia, lymphoma, and cervical cancers are not uncommon. Death often results from one or a combination of these complications in a person with AIDS.

The newest way to monitor treatment effectiveness for HIV patients is to follow the patient's viral load. This measurement uses complicated biological tests to see how much virus is in circulation. If viral load is low, then the treatment is working well to keep the virus suppressed. If viral load is high, the patient may have developed resistance to the present treatment. New tests can even measure whether the virus is susceptible to certain drugs.

What Treatments Are Available for AIDS?

Despite the massive efforts being put forth to save people infected with HIV, there currently is no cure for AIDS. What follows is a very brief summary of the types of treatments in common use:

- **Antiviral drugs** Antiviral drugs inhibit replication of HIV. The first and best studied of these is AZT, or zidovudine. This class of drugs does not cure HIV, but it has shown positive short-term effects on AIDS patients. Some antiviral drugs also have significant toxic side effects, which limit their use.

  There are other antiviral drugs similar to zidovudine. Use of them in combination with zidovudine may prevent the virus from developing a drug resistance. One of these drugs, lamivudine, or 3TC, when combined with AZT seems to make the virus sensitive to treatment again.

A new class of antivirals became available in early 1996: protease inhibitors. These drugs work by blocking an enzyme (protease) unique to the HIV virus. Without this enzyme, maturation and replication of the virus is prevented. Therefore, when used in combination with the antivirals mentioned previously, protease inhibitors reduce the amount of infectious virus in circulation. These medicines prolong survival of people with AIDS if used in combination.

A recent study has shown that taking zidovudine during pregnancy and delivery, and then giving the drug to the newborn, will greatly reduce the chances a baby will acquire HIV from its mother. Conducted at several universities, the study showed that taking AZT reduced the risk of infection of the newborn from 25% to 8%. This provides a very good reason to test pregnant women for HIV. Cesarean section may reduce this percentage even further.

D. E. Shapiro et al., "Risk factors for perinatal human immunodeficiency virus transmission in patients receiving zidovudine prophylaxis; Pediatric AIDS Clinical Trials Group Protocol 076 Study Group," *Obstetrics and Gynecology* 94(6): 897–908 (1999).

- **Symptomatic therapy** A long and growing list of medications and treatments are used to treat the numerous complaints of AIDS patients as they progress through the disease.

- **Prophylactic treatment** Antibiotics such as co-trimoxazole have been very successful (95%) in preventing Pneumocystis pneumonia. Other drugs such as clarithromycin can help prevent fever and weight loss due to Mycobacterium avium, a tuberculosis-like illness common to AIDS patients.

- **Immune system stimulants** Interferon and other drugs attempt to boost the failing immune system and ward off infection. The results with this approach to treatment so far have been disappointing.

- **Alternative treatments** Unproven therapies not endorsed by the U.S. Food and Drug Administration are often available through underground networks. These networks are fueled by the panic among some people stricken with AIDS who see others dying despite mainstream treatments. Unfortunately, many unsafe drugs and practices are offered to the public; these can cause great harm or even death. Examples of unproven treatments are coffee and freon enemas, ozone treatments, and megadose mineral and vitamin therapies.

How Do My Partner and I Keep from Getting AIDS?

Prevention of the HIV infection is the only safe approach for avoiding AIDS. The time may come when we can indefinitely prolong the lives of those who have AIDS, as well as offer them a reasonably good quality of life. That time has not come yet, and no one is certain when or if it will.

We will not focus on the details of transmission of the HIV virus by routes such as intravenous drug use and blood transfusion. There are a number of excellent books that can provide detailed information about the risks of these avenues of infection. In *Your Guy's Guide to Gynecology*, we concentrate on the growing problem of sexual transmission of HIV.

AIDS has quickly become the most deadly sexually transmitted disease of all. As you can see from the statistics at the beginning of this chapter, the rate of transmission of this deadly illness through heterosexual contact is increasing rapidly. Everyone who is sexually active, or hopes to be, needs to be concerned about the possibility of getting HIV from a sexual partner. Recall that most people who have the infection have no symptoms for several years, and many are unaware they have it.

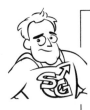

Supportive Guy Recommends:

1. The safest sex is no sex—abstinence. Massage, hugging, mutual masturbation, and closed-mouth kissing are safe substitutes for intercourse.

2. Enjoy a mutually monogamous relationship with someone who is HIV negative. Abstain from intercourse or use a condom for the first six months (in order to know with certainty whether you are HIV negative, you both would require testing six months after your last possible exposure to HIV).

3. If your partner is other than monogamous, use a condom with spermicide every time you have sex. See the recommendations for condom use at the end of Chapter 4.

4. Do not have sex with prostitutes. Many have been found to be HIV positive.

5. Do not have sex with people from high-risk groups (intravenous drug users, those with multiple sexual partners) or people who are infected with HIV. If you do, use a condom with spermicide and avoid contact with their body fluids.

6. Avoid types of sexual activity likely to tear the genital tissues (e.g., penile-anal intercourse).

7. Condoms are recommended for oral-penile sex unless both partners are known to be HIV negative.

8. Keep your partner safe. Do not use intravenous drugs, or if you do, seek help from a treatment program. Never share needles with another user.

9. Women can use a female condom, or "vaginal pouch," if their partners refuse to wear a condom, but this is not an adequate substitute.

Notes about Condom Use

- Don't use petroleum jelly; it makes condoms dissolve!
- Polyurethane condoms can be used in place of latex condoms for those who are allergic to latex.
- Latex condoms are preferred over the natural skin type because they are better at preventing transmission of HIV.
- There is now good evidence that even latex condoms are not completely effective at preventing HIV:

A study in 1987 showed that 17% of women whose partners were HIV infected acquired the disease themselves despite consistent and proper use of latex condoms. Another study in 1993 showed condoms to be only 69% effective in preventing HIV in heterosexual couples.

M. A. Fischl et al., "Evaluation of heterosexual partners, children and household contacts of adults with AIDS," *Journal of the American Medical Association* 257: 640 (1987); H. S. Weinstock et al., "Factors associated with condom use in high-risk heterosexual population," *Sexually Transmitted Diseases* 20: 14 (1993).

If your partner is from a high-risk group, or may have had a partner who was, remember abstinence as an option until HIV testing can *prove* your partner is uninfected.

Admittedly, HIV infection is a difficult subject for anyone to confront. It is even more awkward to discuss this disease as a couple, especially early in a relationship when it is most important. We strongly urge you to talk about AIDS and other STDs with each other *before* you become intimate. An open and honest conversation about your prior sexual history and possible exposures is an unfortunate necessity at this time in our society. Although it may be uncomfortable, this type of communication shows respect and caring for your partner and will help to build a strong relationship.

POST TEST

1. Only men can get AIDS.
   T or F

2. An ELISA test of the blood is enough to diagnose someone with HIV infection.
   T or F

3. A flu-like illness can be the first sign of HIV infection.
   T or F

4. AIDS is a form of cancer.
   T or F

5. Abstinence from sex will help prevent HIV infection.
   T or F

6. Condoms are recommended for oral sex to reduce the spread of HIV.
   T or F

7. A new condom should be used for each act of intercourse to help prevent the spread of HIV (and decrease the risk of pregnancy).
   T or F

8. Petroleum jelly is the best lubricant to use with a condom.
   T or F

9. Intravenous drug use can increase the risk of acquiring HIV, especially if needles are shared.
   T or F

10. Having only one sexual partner and talking honestly about prior sexual practices can help reduce the spread of HIV.
    T or F

Key: 1. F   2. F   3. T   4. F   5. T   6. T   7. T   8. F   9. T   10. T

ATTACK OF THE KILLER HORMONES **6**

"Honey, I'm home!"

(No answer.)

"Honey . . . ?"

(Silence.)

Slowly he walks through the house, becoming increasingly alarmed as he observes signs of an apparent struggle: beds unmade, papers strewn about, dirty dishes everywhere. Their usually tidy house seems to have been visited by an indoor tornado.

At last he finds her, hunched silently in front of the TV, hands clutching a near-empty Doritos bag. With tears streaming from her eyes, she stares at a Melrose Place rerun and continues to ignore his presence.

"Hi. Are you okay? What happened here today?" he asks with concern.

"WHAT DO YOU MEAN, WHAT HAPPENED?!" she snaps.

"I mean, the house looks terrible, and you look . . . upset!"

(Silence.)

(More silence.)

"YOU NEVER REALLY LOVED ME!" she blurts.

"Honey, of course I love—"

"YOU THINK I'M FAT!!" She sobs openly.

(Even more silence.)

He suddenly remembers an urgent home-repair project, requiring an immediate trip to the hardware store. He exits, stage left.

The apparent struggle that precipitated this slightly dramatized scene was a hormonal phenomenon known as PMS, or the premenstrual syndrome. For those women who have it, and for many men who have been exposed to someone with it, the lesson is clear: PMS is real, and it can be quite severe.

A very different but often troubling hormonal event in women's lives is known as the menopause. Occurring in women at, on average, the age of 51, the menopause heralds the end of a woman's reproductive years. The physical and psychological changes brought on by falling estrogen levels can be just as difficult to manage as PMS.

So what's a guy to do? Suddenly outflanked by a partner who seems to have become a somewhat less kinder, gentler person, many men retreat to the relative safety of their garage. Here, they may find themselves "fixing that damn toaster" for several evenings, or changing the oil on both cars and then the lawnmower. And then offering the same service to the neighbors. Some desperadoes even sneak a few personal articles out of the house in an attempt to set up temporary residence by the Weedwacker.

These "coping strategies" may work briefly, but they eventually fall short of fulfilling the needs of either partner. We suggest instead that, when faced with such a situation, you read this chapter, "The Attack of the Killer Hormones." In the first section, you'll find out what PMS is, what symptoms it causes, and how it's diagnosed. We follow with a detailed discussion of the available treatments—and there are many. This section ends with specific recommendations for you if your partner has PMS, and our own "Top Ten List of Things We Don't Recommend You Say to a Woman with PMS." Memorize this list and then destroy it.

The second section of this chapter covers the menopause. To paraphrase one of our patients, "These aren't the *golden* years—I call these the *rusty* years!" Even if your partner hasn't reached this stage in her life, you probably know someone who has. In this section, you'll find out what the menopause is, and how it affects women both physically and mentally. We review standard treatments such as hormone replacement therapy with estrogen and progesterone, newer medications like etidronate and tamoxifen, and alternative treatments like motherwort and dong quai (!). Finally, Supportive Guy chimes in with valuable hints for how to behave with someone who's going through the change.

Although it may not be a summer blockbuster, "The Attack of the Killer Hormones" is filled with useful stuff for men who want to be supportive of their mates. Particularly if they don't know how to fix toasters.

GUY-Q TEST

1. The term PMS means:
   a. peri-menopausal symptoms.
   b. premenstrual syndrome.
   c. a difficult time of the month for your partner.
   d. b and c.

2. PMS:
   a. commonly occurs in women in their 30s and 40s.
   b. is *not* responsive to changes in diet and exercise.
   c. affects men as well as women.
   d. all of the above.

3. Women with PMS may complain of:
   a. depression and/or aggression.
   b. breast tenderness.
   c. fluid retention and bloating.
   d. all of the above.

4. Symptoms of PMS:
   a. usually improve with the start of a menstrual period.
   b. are identical for each woman who has PMS.
   c. never change over time.
   d. all of the above.

5. PMS can be treated with:
   a. daily exercise.
   b. vitamin B_6.
   c. birth control pills.
   d. chips, chocolate, and diet sodas.
   e. a, b, and c; d is the claim of a desperate woman.

6. Treatments for complaints arising during the menopause include:
   a. estrogen.
   b. exercise and calcium.
   c. bisphosphonates (e.g., alendronate).
   d. all of the above.

7. Hot flashes or flushes are caused by:
   a. drinking hot coffee or soup too fast.
   b. overexercising.
   c. a drop in estrogen levels in women.

8. Which of the following may occur with the menopause?
   a. vaginal dryness
   b. insomnia
   c. no more menstrual periods
   d. all of the above

9. A blood test that may be helpful in diagnosing the menopause includes testing for the:
   a. thyroid-stimulating hormone level.
   b. follicle-stimulating hormone level.
   c. hot flash–stimulating hormone level.

10. Menopause is:
    a. a time when sudden sensations of extreme heat of the upper chest and face, called hot flashes, can awaken a woman from sleep.
    b. a popular topic of television talk shows.
    c. a time when a woman's risk of heart disease and stroke may increase significantly.
    d. all of the above.

Key: 1. d   2. a   3. d   4. a   5. e   6. d   7. c   8. d   9. b   10. d

PREMENSTRUAL SYNDROME

What Is PMS?

A standard definition of the premenstrual syndrome is "the regular occurrence of premenstrual (before the menstrual period) physical and/or emotional symptoms of sufficient severity to disrupt daily activities of work or lifestyle."

You will recall from Chapter 1 (see "The Menstrual Cycle") that there are two parts of the menstrual cycle before the period starts: the follicular phase, when the egg develops in the ovary, and the luteal phase (after ovulation), when the uterine lining is prepared for pregnancy. The luteal or premenstrual phase is when PMS symptoms occur. Progesterone and estrogen levels initially rise and then fall during the luteal phase, if no pregnancy occurs.

What Symptoms Does PMS Cause?

PMS takes as many forms as the women who suffer it. For some, the physical symptoms predominate: breast tenderness, bloating, headaches, generalized swelling, and uterine cramps. Other women experience emotional changes: crying spells, anxiety, clumsiness, loss (or increase) in sex drive, depression, lethargy, anger, or aggression. Most have some combination of physical and emotional effects. Those listed above are just the most common; more than 150 different symptoms have been attributed to PMS.

Because of the wide variety of symptoms of women with PMS, some attempts are now being made to standardize the diagnosis. The following criteria have been suggested:

- cyclic premenstrual symptoms
- increase in severity of symptoms as the menstrual period approaches
- relief that comes with the menstrual flow
- at least 7 to 10 days per month free from symptoms
- three consecutive cycles affected
- symptoms significantly interfere with work/social activities or relationships with other people

Although most women have some premenstrual symptoms, the great majority are not disabled by them. When PMS is severe, however, it can damage relationships, careers, and families. One source estimates that between two and five million women in the United States have severe premenstrual syndrome (known as Premenstrual Dysphoria Disorder), or about five percent of those women having regular cycles.* Having seen many patients with significant PMS, we know it can be both physically and emotionally distressing. Beyond the physical discomforts, many women feel guilty about the way they treat the people around them during their PMS, but find it difficult to stop themselves. Reassuringly, it is rare for women to become physically violent.

What Causes PMS?

This is one of those opportunities where we (doctors) could stand tall in our white coats and throw a lot of meaningless information your way. The truth is, nobody knows what causes PMS. There are many theories, and maybe there is some truth in them; maybe there isn't. Popular theories include:

- neurotransmitter dysfunction (neurotransmitters are the chemicals that allow cells in the nervous system to "talk" to each other)
- progesterone deficiency
- prostaglandin imbalance (prostaglandins are powerful chemicals that affect the pelvic organs)
- fluid retention (actually, this is a common symptom of PMS)
- vitamin deficiency
- mineral deficiency
- psychosomatic illness (or "It's all in her head.")

Neurotransmitters, serotonin in particular, seem the most promising candidates at the present time.

---

*M. Steiner et al., "Canadian Fluoxetine/Premenstrual Dysphoria Collaboration Study Group; Fluoxetine in the treatment of premenstrual dysphoria," *New England Journal of Medicine* 332(23): 1529–34 (1995).

How Do You Diagnose PMS?

The diagnosis of PMS is primarily made by talking with a woman about her symptoms. There are no blood tests, physical findings, or psychiatric profiles that are diagnostic. Often, we will ask a patient to record her symptoms as they occur for three months and bring in this "symptom diary." Many times we find that her symptoms are not actually related to her menstrual cycles, or are not repetitive—suggesting a problem other than PMS. Close to 30% of women who think they have PMS have some other disorder. One in four have something else in addition to PMS, such as thyroid gland dysfunction or depression. It is sometimes helpful also to have a co-worker or significant other monitor a woman's symptoms and behavior, for a different perspective.

In addition to determining if her symptoms fit the description of PMS, the doctor must also get a general medical and gynecologic history. Information about current health problems, menstrual history, and work and marital/social situations, in addition to a physical examination, are helpful. Certain physical or emotional problems, medications, drug abuse, or interpersonal problems can either masquerade as PMS or exaggerate its effects.

Is There a Cure for PMS?

In *The Cherry Orchard*, A. P. Chekhov wrote: "If many remedies are prescribed for an illness, you may be certain that the illness has no cure." He may have been thinking about PMS.

There are many treatments for PMS, but there is no cure. This is probably due to our incomplete understanding of its cause, and the many different ways PMS can affect women. At present, treatment is individualized for each woman with PMS.

What Can Be Done to Help a Woman with PMS?

For women with mild to moderate PMS symptoms, the following approach is often used to start therapy:

General Measures (Nonpharmacological)

1. **Dietary Recommendations** During the second half of the cycle, a woman with PMS should eat frequent small meals and replace sweets (chocolate) with complex carbohydrates (vegetables, grains) and a more balanced diet. Calcium, 1 gm./day throughout the month, has recently been shown to help if taken for three or more months. Caffeine in all of its forms (coffee, tea, chocolate, cocoa) may cause headaches and worsen breast tenderness and therefore should be avoided. The woman should reduce or eliminate alcohol, which may worsen fatigue and depression. Salty foods cause water retention, so they are best avoided before her period.

2. **Exercise** Daily aerobic exercise during the luteal phase is a good way to deal with anxiety, anger, and depression. It is also believed to decrease menstrual cramps.

3. **Stress reduction** She can work on reducing stress at work and/or at home throughout the month. Learning some relaxation techniques, practicing conflict resolution, and taking time out for herself will lead to overall less anxiety and therefore less trouble during PMS times.

Following these recommendations for two to four months will be very helpful for most women.

For women who continue to have distressing symptoms, or for women with severe PMS, the following treatments have been used with some success:

Symptom-Specific Treatments

1. **Vitamin B$_6$** A woman with PMS may be treated with vitamin B$_6$: 50 to 200 milligrams per day, starting one day before her symptoms begin. This has been reported to help with breast tenderness, depression, irritability, bloating, and headaches. The dose should not exceed 500 milligrams per day because of potential toxicity.

2. **Oil of evening primrose** Three grams per day of oil of evening primrose, a plant extract rich in essential fatty acids, beginning at midcycle, has been reported to decrease swelling and breast tenderness in some patients. Four months of treatment may be required to determine if it is working.

3. **Diuretics** Spironolactone and other diuretics have been used to help with bloating, fluid retention, and breast tenderness. Some of these prescription medicines may decrease serum potassium, which can cause heart problems. Diuretics should be used sparingly, and only while under the care of a physician.

4. **Oral contraceptives** Oral contraceptives (OCs) often cause significant improvements in PMS symptoms. "The pill" suppresses ovulation as well as the monthly fluctuation of estrogen and progesterone levels, which may play a role in the genesis of PMS. A small number of women, however, actually *develop* PMS while on "the pill." If a woman is currently on OCs and experiencing PMS, she should consult her doctor. Switching pills or making diet and lifestyle changes may help.

5. **Progesterone** The majority of good scientific studies have failed to show progesterone works better than a placebo at alleviating symptoms of PMS. Some patients, however, say it saved their lives. For them, progesterone seems to relieve depression and fluid retention. One notable drawback to progesterone therapy: it is often given by injection or vaginal suppository. A new oral progesterone is becoming more available, and research is ongoing to develop a nasal ointment containing progesterone.

6. **Bromocriptine** Bromocriptine, a prescription medicine, inhibits the release of prolactin, a pituitary hormone that stimulates the breast. Some patients with breast swelling and tenderness find relief with this drug. Side effects are nausea and low blood pressure (which can cause dizziness).

7. **Antidepressants** In keeping with the current trend of trying fluoxetine hydrochloride (trade name Prozac) on everything and everyone (including household pets), researchers have looked into the effects of antidepressants on women with PMS. Preliminary evidence suggests certain antidepressants may be helpful in controlling food cravings and improving mood. However, 40% of patients in one study did not experience improvement in their PMS, and 42% dropped out because of intolerable side effects.*

*M. Steiner et al., Canadian Fluoxetine/Premenstrual Dysphoria Collaboration Study Group, "Fluoxetine in the treatment of premenstrual dysphoria," *New England Journal of Medicine* 332(23): 1529–34 (1995).

Caution: Antidepressants may be helpful in some situations, but they may also remove the desire to address problems in people's lives. For example, if your lousy marriage no longer makes you depressed, why fix it? For the best long-term results, these medications should probably be combined with some form of psychotherapy.

8. **Other hormonal therapies** Danazol, a synthetic anti-estrogen compound, has been used to treat PMS. It has fallen into disfavor because of its masculinizing side effects—deepening of the voice, weight gain, acne, and other unpleasantries. The Gn RH analogs (lupreolide acetate and nafarelin), which temporarily shut down the ovaries, are also being studied for use in PMS.

Again, most women experience significant relief from their PMS by adhering to the general recommendations (as stated above) for at least three months. Successful treatment requires long-term compliance with diet, exercise, and lifestyle changes, and for some, use of prescription medications. PMS is not a simple problem, nor does it have an easy solution. The good news is that you can help—at least according to Supportive Guy:

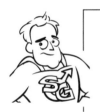

If Your Partner Has PMS

1. Help out more around the house during her PMS times. Whatever you can do to relieve her daily stress will decrease her suffering.
2. Be understanding of her moods. Despite her best efforts, she may not be able to completely control them at this time of the month.
3. Ask her how she's feeling. Ask her what you can do to help. Listen patiently. Realize she probably feels guilty when she overreacts.
4. Encourage her to exercise. Whether it's by offering to exercise with her, or doing things to help her so she has time to go, daily vigorous exercise will help her feel better.
5. Help her watch her diet during this time. Watch *your* diet, too: Don't eat a big bowl of buttery popcorn in front of her during the week before her period.

(continued)

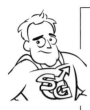

6. Pay attention to her progress as she's being treated. Her doctor may ask you to record your observations of her behavior because you may be able to be more objective.

Just as important as any of the treatments for women with PMS is the understanding and encouragement they receive from their partners at home. We cannot stress this point enough: if a woman knows her significant other understands her difficulty in managing her PMS, it really helps to reduce her guilt and suffering.

In closing, we'd like to remind you that what you say around your partner is just as important as what you do:

TOP TEN LIST OF THINGS WE DON'T RECOMMEND YOU SAY TO A WOMAN WITH PMS

10. Hey, what happened to that big bag of chips we had?

9. Let's rent that new movie *Honey, I Shot the Kids!*

8. Surprise! I invited the boss and his wife over for dinner tonight.

7. The chain saw is in the garage. Why?

6. Hey, those jeans used to be real loose on you, didn't they?

5. I'll arm wrestle you for the last Dove Bar!

4. Honey, you have to stop using that Nordstrom card!

3. I told my mother she could come live with us, okay?

2. Yes, of course I have a life insurance policy. Why?

1. Aw, c'mon—that PMS stuff is all in your head!

THE MENOPAUSE

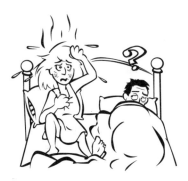

A dark suburban bedroom, late at night. Silence fills the air, save for the relaxed breathing of a middle-aged man. The woman lying beside him, her face beet red and twisted anxiously, suddenly throws off the covers with an exasperated sigh. Her husband awakens with this, but knows better than to question what has become a nightly ritual in their home.

She doesn't sleep; she complains about the heat in the dead of winter; she won't make love because she's "too dry" or "too tired." She cries when he asks why; she cries when he asks anything.

"Who is this person who has taken my wife's body?" he wonders. The theft that occurred just a few months before stole the joy from both of them, and was slowly twisting her into a shadow of her former self.

Sound like a bad B movie? Actually, scenes just like this are played out thousands of times each day by real people, suffering real anxiety, frustration, and fear. The criminal here, the "evil" that attacked this couple, is the menopause. It is not a disease, but a normal event in a woman's life.

What Is the Menopause?

The menopause, also known as the "change of life," is defined by our medical textbooks as one year after the end of a woman's menstrual periods. It occurs on average at age 51. Approximately 25% of women will experience it before the age of 45; the best predictor for an individual woman is the age at which her mother and sisters entered the menopause. A common exception to this occurs when a woman has both ovaries removed: "Surgical" menopause will occur then, regardless of her age.

With increasing life expectancy, a woman today can expect to live a full one-third of her life *after* the "change."

How Do You Know a Woman Has Entered the Menopause?

Menopause occurs when the ovaries stop working. Despite the hormonal commands from the pituitary, the ovaries refuse to produce an egg or as much of their hormones, estrogen and progesterone. A common test for the diagnosis of menopause is to check the blood level of a pituitary hormone, the follicle-stimulating hormone (FSH).

Follicle–stimulating hormone is one of the primary hormones that stimulate the ovaries. The pituitary gland sends out more FSH if it senses low estrogen levels, as happens with the menopause. FSH levels in the blood are therefore high when a woman enters the menopause (usually!).

What Symptoms Does the Menopause Cause?

With the fall in estrogen levels caused by the menopause, many women experience some or all of the following:

- absent menstrual cycles
- hot flashes or flushes
- dryness of the vagina
- psychological symptoms

Absent menstrual cycles are a predictable result of the end of ovarian function. When the ovaries are no longer making much estrogen and progesterone or producing an egg, no lining in the uterine cavity (the endometrium) develops. The loss of menses may be sudden, or may take the form of irregular, unpredictable vaginal bleeding for a few years while the ovaries convert from "part-time" to "unemployed." It cannot be stressed too much how taxing it is for our patients to endure the months of uncertain and often extremely heavy flow during the time just before the menopause, called the perimenopause. Adding to this tension is the fact that these irregular bleeding episodes can be a sign of another problem, uterine cancer.

Hot flashes or flushes occur during the menopause, along with the falling estrogen levels, although what causes them is unclear. Approximately 80% of menopausal women will complain of this sudden flushing of the skin of the face, neck, and/or chest, and a feeling of intense warmth. Four out of five women will endure these sensations for more than a year, and almost half of all menopausal women will experience them for more than five years. The flushes last from a few seconds to a few minutes, and occur more often at times of stress or at night. If they disrupt sleep on a regular basis, they may contribute to chronic sleep deprivation. Other associated symptoms include nausea, dizziness, heart palpitations, headaches, and sweating.

Dryness of the vagina is another result of lower estrogen levels. Regardless of whether the male partner notices this change, the discomfort and diminished sensitivity can make sex much less appealing to women. All of the reproductive tissues in the genital area lose some of their blood flow with the withdrawal of hormones, and begin to atrophy, or age: the clitoris shortens and the bladder and urethra may lose some of their support—incontinence (involuntary loss of urine) may result. Even the breast tissues change with the decrease of estrogen: they become softer and less erect, and the nipples respond less to stimulation.

Psychological symptoms may be a major part of the change of life. Fatigue, nervousness, headaches, insomnia, forgetfulness, depression, irritability, dizziness, and difficulty concentrating are commonly reported. Many of these symptoms are related at least in part to lack of sleep because of hot flashes and will therefore improve if the hot flashes are adequately treated.

Now for the "silent but deadly" department: The above symptoms are difficult to ignore for most women at this time of their lives. Two other major changes at this time go unnoticed, because of their lack of symptoms, but are at least as important: increased cardiovascular disease and osteoporosis.

A doubling of the risk of heart attacks and strokes occurs with the fall of estrogen levels associated with the menopause. This is believed to be caused by changes in cholesterol levels and also the loss of estrogen's beneficial effect on the heart and blood vessels. During their 40s, women have one-half the rate of cardiovascular mortality as their male counterparts. Once they enter their 50s, the rate increases and becomes equivalent to that of men.

Contrary to what you might think, *10 times* more women die of cardiovascular disease than from breast cancer each year in the United States.

Taking estrogen after menopause appears to reduce the risk of cardiovascular death by a full 50%.

A steady decline in bone mass also begins as soon as estrogen levels fall. This silent process is undetectable by common X-ray exams until well into osteoporosis's progression. Left unchecked, osteoporosis leads to an increased risk of fractures. Almost 25% of all women fracture their hips by the age of 90; 80% of these fractures can be attributed to osteoporosis. Fifteen percent of these women will die from complications of broken hips within three months. Wrist fractures and shrinkage of the spine (average spine shrinkage is two and a half inches), the dowager's hump, are the result of osteoporosis as well.

A Note About Bone Density Testing

Since standard X-rays aren't sensitive enough to detect the early changes leading to osteoporosis, new techniques have been developed. The "gold standard" for bone density testing is the DEXA scan, which stands for dual-energy X-ray absorb-tiometry. Use of this test, or another called quantitative ultrasound, allows detection of bone loss before it reaches dangerous levels.

We don't routinely recommend bone mineral density testing for our patients because it's usually unnecessary. Some women, however, may benefit from these tests: those unsure about taking HRT, those who can't take estrogen in any form, and women considering an alternate form of osteoporosis prevention.

Once treatment has begun, bone mineral density testing is usually not repeated. For those women who choose not to treat their bone loss, we may repeat the study in two years.

Risk factors for osteoporosis are a slender build, white or Asian race, smoking, a sedentary (inactive) lifestyle, a family history of osteoporosis, early loss of ovarian function, no childbearing, and chronic steroid therapy.

Protective characteristics include obesity, having more than one child, a muscular build, black race, and prolonged birth control pill use.

Avoidable risks are lack of exercise, smoking, decreased calcium intake, alcoholism, excess caffeine intake, and estrogen deficiency.

As if all this weren't enough, a woman's sex drive often decreases with the arrival of the menopause.

If all this sounds like a pretty unhappy picture, you're getting it right. Thankfully, there is much that she, her doctor, and you can do.

What Treatments Are Available for the Menopause?

Although it's not all that simple, one step in treating many of these symptoms is to give back *some* of the estrogen that has been lost with the menopause. In relative terms, estrogen replacement therapy (ERT) replaces only about 25% of the ovaries' normal production before the menopause. Even this small amount of hormone, however, restores much of the lost quality of life to many menopausal women, and may significantly prolong their lives.

Estrogen is not a panacea for women in the menopause. As women—as well as men—enter middle age, living a healthy lifestyle becomes increasingly important. Specifically, this means eating a balanced diet, exercising frequently, and avoiding smoking and excessive alcohol intake. Obesity and a high-stress life become even more dangerous, and other health problems such as diabetes must be managed well. Women must also pay attention to having an adequate calcium intake.

Estrogen taken without progesterone seems to increase the risk of uterine cancer by overstimulating the endometrial living. Therefore, estrogen is almost always prescribed with a synthetic progesterone (progestin) in order to eliminate this risk. Women who have had a hysterectomy (surgical removal of the uterus) do not need a progestin. When both hormones are given together, the treatment is referred to as hormone replacement therapy, or HRT.

Most women are candidates for HRT. Some women with a history of certain medical problems or cancers cannot use estrogen because of an increased probability of complications. Rarely, women cannot tolerate the side effects of the hormones.

Before the decision is made to begin HRT, each woman should know both the risks and the potential benefits, and should discuss them with her doctor.

Risks of Hormone Replacement Therapy

The risks of hormone replacement therapy include the following:

1. **Gallbladder disease**   Estrogen increases the risk of having painful gallstones; adding a progestin (synthetic progesterone) to the treatment adds additional risk. However, the chance of developing this complication is small.

2. **Cancer of the endometrium**   Long-term use of estrogen without progesterone can significantly increase the risk of cancer of the endometrium (uterine lining). As mentioned previously, prescribing a progestin with the estrogen actually lowers the risk of cancer of the endometrium to less than or equal to that of women who take no hormones. Current estimates place the risk of developing cancer of the uterus at *less than one percent per year* when on standard HRT.

3. **Breast cancer**   Estimates as high as one in eight have now been published for the chance that a woman living to age 85 will develop breast cancer in her lifetime. It's currently unproven whether the low doses of estrogen used in HRT are enough to significantly increase this risk. Current evidence suggests that there might be some small increased chance of breast cancer in women who have taken estrogen for several years.

   Each woman should consult with her health care provider about her own specific risk. Mammography, breast self-exams, and regular checkups are mandatory for menopausal women, whether they are taking hormones or not.

Benefits of Hormone Replacement Therapy

The benefits of hormone replacement therapy include the following:

1. **Decrease in hot flashes**   In the majority of women on low-dose HRT, hot flashes are decreased or eliminated.

2. **Improved lubrication and health of the genital tissues** Over the course of three to nine months, an improvement in vaginal lubrication and elasticity can be appreciated. The impact on a couple's sexual satisfaction is often significant. Not uncommonly, bladder control improves as well.

3. **Improved psychological well-being** Women usually report improved psychological well-being within a few weeks after starting hormone replacement. Sleeping patterns begin to normalize and hot flashes decrease. This is accompanied by other signs of general improvement in mental and physical functioning.

4. **Halted osteoporosis** Low-dose HRT, when accompanied by regular weight-bearing exercise and supplemental calcium (1,000 milligrams per day), should halt osteoporosis. Exercise and calcium alone, even in large amounts, are not sufficient to prevent osteoporosis. Vitamin D, 400 IU/day, is also recommended for women deficient in Vitamin D.

5. **Cardiovascular mortality returned to premenopausal levels** Estrogen causes an increase in HDL cholesterol (good cholesterol) and a decrease in LDL cholesterol (bad cholesterol). Taking standard doses of estrogen causes a 50% reduction in the risk of cardiovascular mortality, which claims more than 350,000 women's lives each year in the United States.

6. **Alzheimer's disease** Recent evidence suggests that estrogen may lower the risk of developing Alzheimer's disease by up to 60%.* Estrogen seems to increase nerve growth factors and blood flow to the brain, leading to improved mental functioning. Other research suggests that this treatment helps maintain verbal memory and the ability to learn new material.

7. **Diabetes** Estrogen appears to lower the risk of developing Type 2 diabetes (adult-onset) and helps with blood sugar control for those who already have the disease.

How Is Hormone Replacement Given?

Once a woman's medical history and physical exam have been completed and a discussion of the risks and benefits has taken

*A. Paganini-Hill and V. W. Henderson, "Estrogen replacement therapy and risk of Alzheimer's disease," *Archives of Internal Medicine* 156: 2213–2217 (1996).

place, the decision to try hormone replacement is often made. Estrogen is most often taken orally in either natural or synthetic forms (Premarin, Ogen, or Estrace are the most common brands in the United States). Although their potencies differ, each brand of estrogen, as prescribed, is believed to be comparable to the others in its effects on a woman's body.

Another way to use estrogen is via a skin patch: the hormone is absorbed directly through the skin. The patches must be changed once or twice a week. The estrogen patch is particularly good for women with certain medical problems (such as high blood pressure), which may be aggravated by taking estrogen orally.

Estrogen is also given, less commonly, via intramuscular injection or in tiny pellets implanted under the skin. Also, gels and creams containing estrogen and/or progesterone (also for skin absorbtion) are being offered by more pharmacies in the United States. This type of hormone delivery may have advantages for some women, although cost is a problem and effectiveness needs to be proven.

Yet another delivery system has been created for estrogen, called Estring. This flexible ring fits snugly into the vagina and releases its hormone slowly into the local tissues. Although it may relieve vaginal dryness and irritation in menopausal women, it won't be of much help against osteoporosis and heart disease.

What Are the Side Effects of Hormone Replacement?

The side effects of HRT are typically mild, but they are worthy of mention. They include breast tenderness, nausea, water retention, return of menstrual-like bleeding, and very slight weight gain (less than five pounds). Often these symptoms disappear shortly after the woman starts the medication, and they can be alleviated by changing the hormone schedule.

The most widely used progestin is medroxyprogesterone acetate (trade name Provera), which can be given cyclically or continuously. Up to 25% of women cannot tolerate the side effects of Provera, which may include bloating, depression, PMS-like symptoms, acne, and breast tenderness. Also, all widely used progestins have a negative effect on a woman's "lipid profile" (cholesterol and triglycerides) and therefore may potentially undo some of the cardiovascular protection of estrogen. Provera remains the first choice of the synthetic progestins because it has the least negative impact in this area. Natural progesterone could be even better, but it's not widely available. The lowest possible effective dose of the progestin, regardless of type, should be used.

Cyclic HRT, the most common schedule for taking hormones, has women take estrogen for 25 to 30 days each month and a progestin for 10 to 13 days. A light period usually follows the end of the progestin cycle. With continuous HRT, women take both estrogen and progestin together every day. The main attraction of this schedule is the possibility of eliminating bleeding. It doesn't always work, especially just after the menopause has occured.

The most unpopular side effect of cyclic HRT for many women is the return of vaginal bleeding. One facet of the menopause that women actually appreciate is the end of their menstrual periods. To be once again faced with the inconvenience and discomfort of vaginal bleeding is unwelcome, and causes many women to stop taking their hormones. Many will never start using estrogen for this reason alone. We must constantly reinforce the value of hormonal therapy to motivate our patients to stay with it. Usually the bleeding decreases over time and will disappear after a few years of hormone replacement. Also, it is important for the couple to realize that the return of her period does not signal the return of her fertility.

When a menopausal woman has vaginal bleeding other than when she's supposed to, she often must have a pelvic exam and a biopsy of the endometrium (uterine lining) performed to rule out cancer.

Endometrial biopsies can be painful, and sometimes they're very difficult to perform. A recent patient of ours was very grateful to have her uterine lining evaluated by ultrasound instead of by biopsy. Recent studies show that cancer can sometimes be excluded if we can demonstrate a thin enough endometrium with ultrasound—and it doesn't hurt!

Ultimately, the proper dosage and schedule of hormonal

therapy must be individualized for each woman who chooses it. Although this may be a nuisance for a short while, there is likely to be a noticeable improvement in well-being for both your partner and your relationship. At the present time, the wealth of experimental data supports the long-term benefits of HRT.

What Other Hormones or Treatments Are Used for the Menopause?

Certain remedies for menopause are aimed at alleviating only one or a few symptoms. A number of nonhormonal medications have been tried in treating hot flashes. Oral clonidine, bromocriptine, and belladonna-ergotamine are somewhat effective but have significant side effects. Research is ongoing to find better nonestrogenic relief for hot flashes.

Many women who have had breast cancer take a medicine called tamoxifen to help prevent a recurrence of their disease. In addition, this drug can help prevent the development of osteoporosis.

However, there has been some concern about tamoxifen's side effects. This medicine may induce cancer of the uterus because it has a mild estrogen effect. Recent research has shown that the risk of this cancer after eight years of tamoxifen use is higher than normal but still quite low. We also know that women with breast cancer have a higher than normal risk for developing uterine cancer, so it is unclear whether the tamoxifen is causing a problem or not. Close follow-up with a gynecologist is important for a woman taking this medicine, and any unexpected bleeding should be reported.

A potential improvement over tamoxifen is raloxifene (trade name Evista). This new medication prevents bone loss and may reduce breast cancer risk without stimulating the uterus. Preliminary data shows a decrease in fractures.* However, Evista use may cause leg cramps, a slight increase in dangerous blood clots, and does not relieve hot flashes.

Another hormone sometimes prescribed for menopausal women is testosterone, the male hormone. There is debate among gynecologists about whether taking a very small dose

*B. Ettinger et al., "Reduction of vertebral fracture risk in postmenopausal women with osteoporosis treated with raloxifene: Results from a 3-year randomized clinical trial; Multiple Outcomes of Raloxifene Evaluation (MORE) Investigators," *Journal of the American Medical Association* 282(7): 11 (1999).

of this hormone can help restore lost libido, or sex drive, in menopausal women. Few scientific studies have been done, but the data seem to indicate that only women having a premature menopause from surgical removal of their ovaries have any real improvement in sex drive with testosterone (though the majority of women who have their ovaries removed don't appear to need it). Care must be used in prescribing this drug because the side effects can be significant: facial hair growth, deepening of the voice, acne, enlargement of the clitoris, liver disease, and weight gain. Thorough counseling and close follow-up with a gynecologist is strongly recommended for any woman considering testosterone.

It should also be kept in mind that testosterone reverses estrogen's positive effect on blood lipids. This effect is very important for reducing cardiovascular mortality, and its loss is no small matter.

Women actually produce a small amount of testosterone, the male hormone, during their reproductive years. Although estrogen levels fall during menopause, testosterone production continues for 3–4 more years.

The prevention of osteoporosis is still important for women who cannot or will not take estrogen. It is crucial for these women to follow the recommendations suggested previously: frequent weight-bearing exercise, good calcium intake, avoidance of smoking, and minimizing caffeine and alcohol intake. Other chemicals that are being studied for use in preventing osteoporosis include parathyroid hormone, fluoride, calcitonin, vitamin D metabolites, and progestins. Some believe that vitamin C intake could help prevent osteoporosis by improving bone density.

A new class of medications being used in the treatment of osteoporosis is the bisphosphonates: etidronate and alendronate. Research has shown that these estrogen-free compounds can help increase bone mass and decrease fractures when used properly. Unfortunately, they are poorly absorbed when taken orally, and women who take them have to follow very specific instructions. Side effects (such as gastric ulcers) can also be a problem. Lastly, women who take etidronate or alendronate for osteoporosis may have to forgo the other significant benefits of estrogen, since they are usually not given together.

Outside of mainstream medicine, some alternative treatments for the menopause seem to benefit some women. Certain chemicals derived from fruits, flowers, and other parts of edible plants, so-called botanical therapies, are a case in point. Some plants, such as black cohosh and blue cohosh, have estrogen-like activity. Other botanicals in use are red raspberry, motherwort, and dong quai.

Like their traditional pharmaceutical counterparts, these botanicals are not without side effects. Black cohosh may cause nausea and vomiting, slow heart rate, and painful uterine contractions. Dong quai and angelica have been noted to cause photosensitivity (light sensitivity) and inhibited blood clotting.

Phytoestrogens are compounds that occur naturally in many foods. They have been shown to have a weak estrogen effect in a woman's body. Examples are soy products, yams, and cereal bran. In their naturally occurring forms, some phytoestrogens need to be eaten in very large quantities to be helpful.

The presence of phytoestrogens may help to explain why vegetarians have a lower risk of coronary heart disease and certain types of cancer. Many studies are currently underway to investigate the effects of these chemicals on both osteoporosis and menopausal symptoms in general.

According to a recent scientific article, hot flashes are far more common in European women (70–80%) than in those from China and Singapore (14–18%). One explanation for this large difference in menopause symptoms is that Asian woment consume far more soy products in their diet.

D. Knight and J. A, Eden, "A review of the clinical effects of phytoestrogens," *Obstetrics and Gynecology* 87(5, part 2): 897–904 (1996).

Nontraditional therapies for menopausal women are intriguing and valuable for some women. We cannot recommend them as enthusiastically as traditional hormone replacement, however, until the necessary research has been done to prove their effectiveness and safety.

Whatever approach your partner chooses in managing her menopause, what you do and say will make a difference.

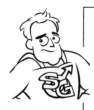

What You Can Do for a Woman Going Through the Menopause

1. Be aware of the changes she's going through, both physically and emotionally. They are often sudden, and because she can't control them, they may be frightening to her. Think of how you'd feel if your body, including your sexual parts, was malfunctioning! Menopause signals the end of her fertility and the beginning of her older age—and that's serious stuff.

2. Talk to her about what she's experiencing. Pat Heim, Ph.D., an acknowledged expert in male-female communication, says it's best to "do a lot of listening. When confronted with a problem, men want to start fixing it and will often start prescribing what she should do. She often feels dismissed by this, and things can go south quickly. Instead, ask a lot of questions: What causes that? Will you need more tests? And don't forget feelings: How are you feeling? Are you scared? What can I do for you? Women deal with emotion by processing, not just talking. Be attentive and let her talk; she'll feel better."

3. Be patient with intercourse. She may take longer to be aroused, and longer to be ready for actual insertion of the penis because of slower lubrication. Even with hormonal therapy, things may not be exactly as they were. Use a lubricant if necessary—they are available without a prescription and can be found in most drug stores. Don't use petroleum jelly—get the newer products; they're much better (for example, Replens, Astroglide, K-Y lubricant).

4. Help her comply with her medications. If she's decided to take hormones, reinforce the decision and help her to remember to take them. Talk to her or her physician if you don't understand or agree with her decision. Get involved—what she does with respect to this issue will affect her health and your life together for a long time.

(continued)

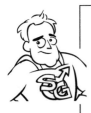

5. Encourage follow-up visits and communication with her health professional. Aside from making necessary adjustments in her medications, she needs regular pap smears and breast exams.

6. Set an example! Get up off the couch! Tuck in that gut, soldier! Quit smoking, quit lecturing, and inspire by example. No excuses. (Perhaps you could also help out more around the house so she has time to exercise.)

POST TEST

1. PMS is a well understood and easily treatable condition.
   T or F

2. Exercise and stress reduction can help reduce the symptoms of PMS.
   T or F

3. Treatment for PMS can be customized for each woman by having her keep a symptom calendar for three months.
   T or F

4. Birth control pills are beneficial for some women with PMS.
   T or F

5. Antidepressant medication has been shown to cure PMS in the majority of cases.
   T or F

6. There are no effective treatments for menopause.
   T or F

7. The changes brought on by menopause can make intercourse painful for some women.
   T or F

8. Osteoporosis is a risk of taking estrogen replacement therapy.
   T or F

9. Hot flashes or flushes can cause insomnia.
   T or F

10. The benefits of taking hormone replacement greatly outweigh the risks for most women.
    T or F

Key: 1. F   2. T   3. T   4. T   5. F   6. F   7. T   8. F   9. T   10. T

COMPLICATED FEMALE STUFF MADE SIMPLE

7

"I appreciate the idea of a book for men. I don't mean to say mean things, but I feel even worse because he doesn't understand my problem."

—Woman interviewed before her hysterectomy

Bladder infections are common. Usually they result in burning and frequent urination for a few days and can be easily treated with a brief course of antibiotics. However, a simple bladder infection can sometimes lead to a severe systemic infection and kidney damage. Did you know that having sex can actually *cause* bladder infections in women?

Any woman who discovers a **breast lump** will likely experience fear. Although most lumps are not cancerous, they require a professional examination and sometimes other testing or even surgery. Are you aware of the risk factors that may put your partner at higher risk of developing breast cancer?

Abnormal Pap smears are often found in young women. Since this test result could indicate a precancerous or cancerous condition of the cervix, abnormal Pap smears may make a woman pretty anxious. Although major surgery is rarely needed, the process of evaluation and treatment can be uncomfortable and frightening. How well do you understand what a woman goes through?

Endometriosis can cause a wide range of problems: pain with intercourse, severe cramps with periods, and even infertility. Surgery is often necessary, sometimes requiring removal of the uterus, tubes, and ovaries. Powerful medications with troubling side effects are often used. Do you understand endometriosis well enough to help your partner?

Uterine fibroids are a common cause of heavy menstrual bleeding and painful periods. They may also cause pelvic pressure, pain with intercourse, frequent urination, or difficulty with bowel movements. Because of all these problems, fibroids are the leading cause of hysterectomy in the United States. If she's deciding whether to have a hysterectomy, have you discussed the alternatives with her?

A word of caution: We're not trying to turn you into a junior gynecologist. However, we've found that problems like bladder infections, endometriosis, and uterine fibroids often cause couples to feel awkward. Without some basic knowledge, you may not know what to say to your mate. A little education, however, can enable you to respond to her in a way that makes your relationship stronger and happier then ever before.

Even if you don't have to deal with any of these issues now, chances are you will someday. So read on, and become an even better partner by learning a little about "complicated female stuff—made simple."

GUY-Q TEST

1. Bladder infections may be diagnosed by:
   a. examining a concentrated urine specimen under the microscope.
   b. checking for bacterial growth in a urine culture.
   c. obtaining a history of burning with urination.
   d. all of the above.

2. Bladder infections may cause the following symptoms:
   a. burning with urination.
   b. frequent voiding of small amounts of urine.
   c. leakage of urine with coughing or sneezing.
   d. no symptoms at all.
   e. all of the above.

3. A breast lump may be caused by:
   a. normal hormonal changes in the breast glands.
   b. a fatty tumor, or lipoma.
   c. an infection during breast-feeding.
   d. breast cancer.
   e. all of the above.

4. Mammograms can pick up breast cancers as small as:
   a. two inches.
   b. half an inch.
   c. one millimeter.

5. For most women, Pap smears should be repeated every:
   a. five years.
   b. one to two years.
   c. six months.

6. Abnormal Pap smears can be found in a woman with:
   a. precancer or cancer of the cervix.
   b. cervical infection.
   c. a normal cervix.
   d. all of the above.

7. Endometriosis is:

   a. diagnosed when endometrial lining is found outside the uterus.

   b. a disease that can cause severe pelvic pain.

   c. sometimes found unexpectedly during pelvic surgery.

   d. all of the above.

8. Endometriosis can be treated by:

   a. oral contraceptive pills.

   b. using medications that raise estrogen levels.

   c. local application of creams.

   d. all of the above.

9. Uterine fibroids are:

   a. a common cause of light bleeding during periods.

   b. cancerous muscular tumors of the uterus.

   c. a common cause of hysterectomy.

10. Fibroids may lead to hysterectomy because:

    a. they can cause heavy menstrual bleeding.

    b. they cause the uterus to grow greatly in size.

    c. they compress the bladder or rectum.

    d. all of the above.

Key: 1. d   2. e   3. e   4. b   5. b   6. d   7. d   8. a   9. c   10. d

BLADDER INFECTIONS

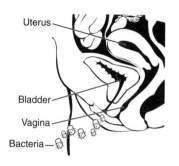

Uterus
Bladder
Vagina
Bacteria

Bladder infections, known in medical circles as UTIs (for urinary tract infections) or cystitis, are a common problem for women. When they cause symptoms like burning with urination, pelvic pain, and fevers, they become a problem that both members of a couple must deal with.

Who Gets Bladder Infections and Why?

Any woman can get a bladder infection, and the same is true for men. Certain groups of women are more likely to get them; they are:

- **Sexually active women** Intercourse, especially frequent intercourse, can lead to more UTIs. Recall from the anatomy section in the first chapter that women have a very short urethra—the tube that empties the bladder. The entrance to the urethra is also right at the top of the vagina. Having sex can easily push some of the normal vaginal bacteria into the bladder, where they don't belong. If enough bacteria get into the bladder, infection often occurs. Now you understand the term for this cause of UTIs: honeymoon cystitis.

- **Pregnant women** High levels of progesterone coupled with compression of the bladder and ureters (the tubes that drain the urine from the kidneys) by the pregnant uterus prevent normal emptying of the urinary tract. This can lead to more infections. Certain events during the delivery process (like draining the bladder with a catheter) also may cause UTIs.

- **Postmenopausal women** Women who have experienced the "change of life" may have more bladder infections, especially if they do not take estrogen. The postmenopausal lower urinary tract becomes thinner and weaker when it's deprived of estrogen. In addition, older women are more likely to suffer from incontinence (involuntary urine loss) and incomplete emptying of the bladder, either of which may lead to infection.

- **The very busy woman** Infrequent emptying of the bladder gives infections more time to get established. Women who are "on the go" have to make time to "go" every few hours or they run the risk of UTIs.

- **Women with chronic medical conditions** Certain neurologic disorders and other diseases such as diabetes increase a woman's chances of getting a bladder infection. This results from an alteration in normal bladder function or from a lowered resistance to infection.

- **Women who undergo pelvic or urologic surgical procedures** Often the bladder may be drained with a catheter before pelvic surgery. Any instrumentation, catheterization, or other manipulation of the bladder temporarily raises the risk of infection.

- **Women with an abnormal urinary tract** An abnormal urinary tract—either congenital (from birth) or caused by a prior injury—can result in more UTIs.

- **Women prone to kidney stones** Kidney stones prevent normal urinary tract emptying, and women with kidney stones may develop more UTIs.

Remember: Any woman can get a bladder infection!

What Symptoms Do Bladder Infections Cause?

The classic symptoms of a bladder infection are burning with urination, more frequent voiding of small amounts of urine, and pelvic pain. However, some women may have no symptoms at all during an episode of cystitis.

At the other extreme, a bladder infection may sometimes result in bloody urine and leakage from the bladder (incontinence), as well as the symptoms mentioned above. If the infection spreads to the bloodstream, a woman may complain of fevers, muscle aches, and fatigue. As the infection progresses, one or both kidneys may become infected as well. This is called pyelonephritis. More aggressive medical treatment is needed if this occurs.

How Are Bladder Infections Diagnosed?

Probably the best tip-off for an episode of cystitis is when a woman with pelvic pain describes burning and/or more frequent urination. The doctor will get very suspicious if the woman is prone to UTIs because of any of the risk factors listed above.

Patients often worry that they have a bladder infection when they notice that their urine is cloudy or has a strong odor. In the absence of other symptoms, this usually just means that the urine is concentrated. The kidneys will conserve water by concentrating the urine if a person is dehydrated.

The diagnosis of cystitis can often be made with a urinalysis, a test in which a drop of urine is examined under the microscope for bacteria and white blood cells (the body's defense against infection). A urine culture may be performed as well. A urine culture can identify the offending bacteria in two to four days and tests it for sensitivity to a number of antibiotics.

Other tests may be run, particularly if the bladder infections are frequent or severe. An intravenous pyelogram (IVP), an X-ray of the kidneys, ureters, and bladder, may be helpful in detecting structural abnormalities of the urinary tract or obstructions to the flow of urine, such as kidney stones. In this test, an intravenous dye is injected into a vein and "lights up" the urinary tract on the X-ray. Cystoscopy, looking into the bladder with a fiber-optic scope, may disclose bladder or urethral abnormalities. A voiding cysto-urethrogram is a test that detects problems with the normal flow of urine.

How Are Bladder Infections Treated?

A typical UTI can be treated with a short course (three to seven days) of oral antibiotics. The choice of antibiotic depends on several factors and is best made by a medical professional. (It is *not* a good idea to check the medicine cabinet to see what antibiotic is left over from your baby's last ear infection.)

It may be necessary to obtain a urine specimen for culture before starting antibiotics. This test will identify both the species of bacteria as well as what antibiotic(s) it's sensitive to. This information may be very helpful in guiding therapy. If the diagnosis of UTI is unclear, the physician may wait for culture results before ordering treatment. If no bacteria grow in the urine culture, usually no treatment is needed.

Critical to the effective treatment of a bladder infection is to continuously empty the bladder. We recommend increasing fluids to two and a half to three liters per day and voiding every two to three hours when awake. This alone can often eradicate an early bladder infection.

Cranberry juice! Drink cranberry juice! What's all this about cranberry juice? Well, it turns out that this stuff probably suppresses growth of bacteria in the bladder by making the urine more acidic. Some scientific studies say that it works; others say it doesn't. Either way, cranberry juice is liquid and therefore promotes emptying the bladder, and that's good for bladder infections.

Pain from bladder infections can be severe. A medicine that works specifically to numb the bladder is called phenazopyridine hydrochloride (trade name Pyridium). It turns the urine a funny orange color, but quickly makes emptying the bladder much less uncomfortable. Once the antibiotics take effect (usually in one to three days), this anesthetic is no longer needed.

Treatment of more severe UTIs, such as a pyelonephritis, may require higher doses of antibiotics, more prolonged treatment, or intravenous antibiotic therapy.

What Serious Consequences Can Result from Bladder Infections?

The typical bladder infection is easily treated once diagnosed. When it progresses to a kidney infection and/or spreads to the bloodstream, major consequences may result. The immediate effects may include fatigue, fevers, and muscle aches. If not adequately treated, the infection may spread to other organs, and a life-threatening infection may occur. Repeated kidney infections may damage the kidneys and/or cause the development of kidney stones.

Pregnant women who have severe urinary tract infections are at risk for the same consequences and, in addition, may have trouble with their pregnancies. Severe infections, dangerous lung problems, and low birth-weight babies (from premature labor and delivery) have resulted from bladder infections that weren't successfully treated.

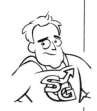

How Can Bladder Infections Be Prevented?

The following steps should help reduce the frequency and severity of UTIs:

- She should completely empty her bladder soon after intercourse to prevent bacteria that have been pushed into the urethra or bladder from establishing an infection.

- Encourage adequate daily fluid intake. She should drink at least eight ounces of water or other fluids every eight hours. Some studies suggest that the regular intake of cranberry juice may be helpful.

- Remind her it's healthy to urinate every few hours and to empty her bladder fully. It's not good to "hold it" if she feels the urge.

- Good hygiene helps. Both you and your partner should keep your genital areas clean. If you are uncircumcised, it's a good idea to clean under the foreskin before sex. For her, it is especially important to wipe from front to back after going to the bathroom. This prevents the movement of bacteria from the rectal area into the vagina.

- If she uses a diaphragm and has frequent UTIs, another method of birth control may be preferable. Diaphragms may make complete emptying of the bladder more difficult.

- Estrogen replacement therapy during menopause may help reverse the thinning of the tissues in the genital area, including the urinary tract. Help her remember to take her estrogen if she's decided to, and it may help reduce UTIs.

- If she has a bladder or urethral problem, or another medical problem that is contributing to her bladder infections, urge her to get effective treatment.

- Her doctor may prescribe prophylactic antibiotics to help reduce UTIs. Help her to remember to take them after sex or as recommended by her doctor.

BREAST LUMPS

What If My Partner Finds a Breast Lump?

To understand breast lumps, you'll need to know a little about the anatomy and physiology of the human breast. The breast is a gland, designed to manufacture and release milk to a newborn infant. During pregnancy, a number of hormones cause massive growth of the glandular tissue within the breast. Milk production occurs within these glands. Networks of glands empty into ducts, which end at the nipples. Suckling at the nipple by the newborn stimulates nerves that cause the secretion of oxytocin, a hormone from the pituitary gland (in the brain). Oxytocin causes the milk to be released from the nipples.

The breast of a woman in the nonpregnant state is primarily made up of fat tissue, with inactive glands, nerves, and blood vessels making up the rest of the structure. The breast sits on the pectoral muscles (see Figure 7.1).

Although it is relatively quiescent, the breast of a nonpregnant woman is still influenced by the cyclic flow of estrogen and progesterone. During the second half of each menstrual cycle (after ovulation), these hormones may stimulate the gland tissue enough to cause breast tenderness, fluid retention, and swelling. These changes are often what women perceive as lumps.

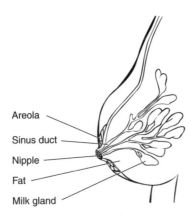

Areola
Sinus duct
Nipple
Fat
Milk gland

Figure 7.1: Breast anatomy

Are Some Women Prone to Develop Breast Cancer?

Overall, one in eight women will develop breast cancer during her lifetime. About 180,000 new cases of breast cancer are diagnosed each year, and approximately 46,000 deaths occur because of the disease, according to the American Cancer Society.

Risk of breast cancer increases with age. At age 30, about 12 in 100,000 women will get the disease. By the age of 50, more than ten times that number of women, 180 in 100,000, will be affected.

A family history of breast cancer may put a woman at increased risk. In particular, if a woman's mother, daughter, or sister has had breast cancer, her risk may be raised significantly. More distant relatives with breast cancer may confer a *slightly* higher risk than that found in the general population.

An area of active research is the genetics of breast cancer inheritance. At the present time, there are at least two gene alterations known to cause a higher than normal risk of developing cancer, known as BrCA1 and 2. If there is a strong family history of breast, colon, or ovarian cancer, or any combination of these, genetic counseling should be pursued. It's important to realize, however, this area of research is very new, and our understanding is still limited.

Women who have never given birth or who started their periods at an early age seem to have a slightly higher risk of breast cancer than women who had children or started their periods later.

Other groups of women at increased risk include:

- those with a prior breast biopsy showing certain types of precancerous tissue;
- those with prolonged exposure to toxic chemicals like insecticides;
- those eating a high-fat diet;
- certain women who smoke cigarettes if they have a particular enzyme deficiency (a deficiency with the "slow acetylators," enzymes that detoxify tobacco-related carcinogens more slowly).

Although it is controversial, some data suggest that taking estrogen during the menopause for 10 years or more may slightly raise a woman's risk of developing breast cancer. There are also studies that show no increased risk with estrogen replacement. On the other hand, we know that heart attacks and strokes are decreased substantially by taking estrogen, and these causes of death kill 10 times more women each year than breast cancer.

Recently it has been shown that some women may decrease their risk of breast cancer by taking an anti-estrogen called tamoxifen. This drug is not without side effects and is known to increase uterine cancer rates slightly. Another medication under investigation, raloxifene, may also help prevent breast cancer without adversely affecting the uterus.

How Are Breast Lumps Examined?

Most breast lumps are *not* cancers. Before actually examining a woman with a breast lump, her doctor will usually ask the following questions:

- How long have you had this?
- Is it tender to the touch?
- Where are you in your menstrual cycle?
- Have you had any discharge or bleeding from your nipples?
- Have you ever had a breast lump before, or any other breast problems?
- Is there any history of breast disease or cancer in your family?

The answers to these questions will help determine how likely it is that the woman has breast cancer—or they may point the way toward other possible diagnoses.

On physical examination, the doctor starts by carefully inspecting both breasts to look for redness, dimpling of the skin, and signs of infection or injury. Each breast is then palpated (felt) for the presence of lumps. The exam is carried out in a systematic way, with each breast checked throughout its circumference. Particular attention is paid to the upper outer quadrant, where the majority of breast gland tissue is concentrated. The area under the arms is checked as well, because breast tissue and lymph nodes extend to that area. We also check for nipple discharge. Bloody nipple discharge may indicate a cancerous condition, whereas milky or clear fluid is usually the result of hormones or medications.

If a lump is cystic (fluid-filled), the doctor may attempt to drain it with a small needle. Usually the lump will shrink or disappear, and the fluid obtained can be tested if necessary for abnormal cells. If the lump feels solid, the doctor may still obtain a small amount of fluid and cells for diagnosis, using a technique called fine needle aspiration. Results from these tests are usually ready in about a week.

What Other Diagnostic Tests Are Used?

The best test for detecting early breast cancer is the mammogram. This is a low-dose X-ray that can detect tumors less than half an inch in diameter—often before a woman or her doctor can feel them. There is no evidence that mammograms are harmful. They can be repeated as needed to help detect early breast cancers.

Although the mammogram is an excellent, lifesaving test for breast cancer, it isn't perfect. Even when properly performed, mammography may miss up to 15% of breast cancers. Therefore mammograms should be supplemented by regular breast exams by a qualified health care practitioner and monthly breast exams by the woman herself. See the Supportive Guy section for recommended mammography intervals.

Ultrasound is often used to help diagnose a woman with a breast lump. An ultrasound unit sends out a directed pulse of sound waves into the tissue in question and uses the echoes sent back to construct an image of the area. This test is particularly useful in differentiating a solid from a cystic lump, which often helps in making a diagnosis.

Another type of breast cancer diagnostic test uses heat sensors to detect tumors. Thermography has not been proven to be as reliable as mammography, at least in part because small tumors (the most important to detect) don't give off much heat at the skin surface.

If the physical exam, mammogram, and ultrasound are not reassuring, it is sometimes necessary to obtain a tissue sample or actually remove the breast lump. Simple biopsy or excisional biopsy, typically done by a general surgeon, obtains enough tissue for the pathologist to make a definitive diagnosis. Further details on these procedures, as well as follow-up, should be discussed with the surgeon performing them.

If It's Not Cancer, What Is It?

As mentioned, most breast lumps, even those found on a mammogram, are not cancer. The following are examples of common, nonmalignant breast problems:

- **Mastalgia**   Tender, swollen breast gland tissue sometimes results from estrogen stimulation. This condition—mastalgia—usually occurs just before a menstrual flow begins and resolves afterward. Up to 60% of women in the menstrual age group may at some time suffer from mastalgia.

- **Fibrocystic breasts**   Many women have thickened fibrous tissue within their breasts that becomes tender and lumpy just before a menstrual period; this is not a disease, but a normal variation of female anatomy. Women with fibrocystic breasts benefit from decreasing the caffeine, chocolate, and fat in their diets, wearing a supportive brassiere, and taking oral contraceptives. Other medications are sometimes used, including diuretics, nonsteroidal anti-inflammatory drugs, danocrine, and tamoxifen. Vitamin E has also been recommended.

 We often see patients who are worried about a tender, swollen, lumpy breast. They are alarmed because the other breast is completely normal. Fibrocystic change, the usual cause, is typically more pronounced on one side.

- **Fibroadenomas**   Fibroadenomas are common, benign (noncancerous) tumors usually found in the breasts of young women. Fibroadenomas are usually removed with a minor surgical procedure to prevent continued growth.

Examples of other, less common benign conditions causing breast lumps are duct ectasia, lipomas, fat necrosis, mastitis, galactocele, superficial thrombophlebitis, and chronic periare-olar abscesses. Their exact definitions are not that important; it's just reassuring to know that many different types of non-cancerous lumps are found in the human breast.

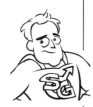

How Can I Help My Partner?

Being the Supportive Guy you are, you want to know how to help promote good breast health for your partner. Aside from offering to check her breasts daily yourself, here are some useful suggestions:

1. **Breast self-exam** This is first because it's most important. Half of all breast cancers are found by the woman herself, and the earlier they're found, the better the chance for cure. Encourage your partner to examine her breasts each month after her period. If she no longer has menstrual periods, she should pick a day that's easy to remember (like the first of the month) and do it then. For specific instructions on how she should perform the breast self-exam, consult her health care provider; numerous pamphlets are also widely available.

2. **Regular exams by a doctor or qualified health professional** As an important supplement to her own breast exams, she should be seen by a trained professional. This person can recommend at what age these exams should be started and how often they should be repeated. Remember that anytime she finds a lump, a breast exam should be done.

3. **Mammograms** We currently recommend that our patients have a mammogram every one to two years beginning at the age of 50 and until the age of 74. They are started earlier if a woman wants to or if there is a risk factor (like a family history of breast cancer). Her doctor should be consulted if there is any question about her risks.

4. **Limiting exposure to environmental toxins** Knowledge about the effects of environmental toxins on the breast is limited, but it seems logical to avoid insecti-cides and to thoroughly wash fruits and vegetables before eating them. We also recommend not breathing the fumes from cleaning agents, fuels, and solvents.

(continued)

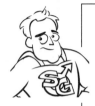

5. **Eat a low-fat diet**   Encourage her to reduce the fat in the foods she eats and to cut back on meat. She can try low-fat or nonfat alternatives (Note: Many food manufacturers replace fat with sugar, which is bad if weight loss is also a goal). She shouldn't drink more than one or two alcoholic drinks per day. There are plenty of benefits for *both* of you in following this advice, so set a good example with your own eating and drinking habits.

6. **If she does find a breast lump, remember the following:**

   a.   It's unlikely to be cancer, but it should be checked.

   b.   Encourage her to express her fears and other feelings to you. Being a good listener is usually enough; you don't have to make it go away.

   c.   Many lumps are just cyclic breast changes caused by hormones and will go away after her period. Discourage her from repeatedly poking and squeezing the lump, as that may slow its disappearance.

ABNORMAL PAP SMEARS

Two patients commented recently about their partners during evaluation of their abnormal pap smears:

"Because of him not being here, I feel like I'm in this by myself. I feel alone, whereas in everything else, we do things together."

—S. T., San Diego, CA

"I know he genuinely cares about me, because he's taken the time to learn about my abnormal pap smear."

—M. M., Brawley, CA

What Is a Pap Smear?

A Pap smear (named after George Papanicolaou, an American anatomist) is a microscopic evaluation of the cells of the cervix. It is performed by gently scraping the cervix with a small wooden spatula, and then using a tiny bottle brush–like instrument in the canal of the cervix. The cells obtained from the two areas are "smeared" on a slide and then sent to a laboratory for interpretation. Trained cytologists and pathologists can detect precancerous changes in individual cells, often allowing a patient to be treated before true cancer of the cervix occurs. Pap smears are necessary because most women will have *no symptoms* from cervical precancer.

Recently, tests have appeared that may improve upon the diagnostic accuracy of the Pap by using new technology. Automated cell screening (e.g., Thin Prep), may be worth the added costs if it proves to be more accurate, i.e., if more abnormal cervices are detected early.

Recall from Chapter 1 (see "Female Anatomy") that the cervix is the open end of the uterus and lies at the top of the vagina. Its opening allows sperm to travel upward into the uterus for fertilization. The cervix also allows passage of menstrual blood out of the uterus each month.

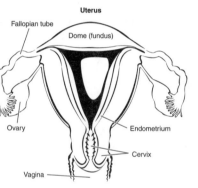

The cervix, like all tissues, is made up of specialized cells and connective tissue. On its surface, the cellular makeup of the cervix is quite complex. One type of cell lining, made up of glands that secrete mucus, meets up with another type that is like the skin of the vagina. During the course of a woman's reproductive life, the skin, or squamous, cells gradually replace part of the glandular tissue. This process of rapid cell division and differentiation is what makes the cervix so prone to cancer.

In addition, the cervix is exposed to sexually transmitted diseases like Human Papilloma Virus (HPV), the venereal wart virus. As many as 30% of sexually active adults may have had exposure to this virus.* Some types of HPV can cause precancerous or cancerous changes to occur on the cervix. This virus is the single biggest reason women have abnormal Pap smears. Other sexually transmitted diseases, including the herpes virus, are not presently believed to cause cancer of the cervix.

---

*R. M. Richart, "Natural history of cervical intraepithelial neoplasia," *Clinical Obstetrics and Gynecology* 10:748 (1967).

Cigarette smoking increases the risk of developing cervical cancer. Carcinogens in smoke are found in high concentration in the mucus made by cervical glands.

If left unchecked, the cervix will be the most common site for female genital cancer—more common than the ovary, uterus, vagina, or vulva. This statement is born out year after year in developing countries, where women don't receive Pap smears. The Pap smear saves thousands of lives each year by detecting precancer which can be successfully treated.

What Is an Abnormal Pap Smear?

Abnormal Pap smears contain cells that are either cancerous, precancerous, or atypical. Various classification schemes have been used over the years to describe the precancerous cells. The current system, called the Bethesda System, was created in 1988. It classifies cells according to the treatment their host is likely to need. Cervical cells are classified as follows (see Figure 7.2):

- **Within normal limits**   Only normal cells are seen.

- **Atypical squamous cells of uncertain significance (ASCUS)**   This classification actually just means the cells are not quite normal, but don't fit into the other groups. The cervix in question may be normal, inflamed, precancerous, or (rarely) cancerous.

- **Low-grade squamous intraepithelial lesion (LGSIL)** This indicates cells that either are infected with HPV (the wart virus) or are mildly precancerous, or both.

- **High-grade squamous intraepithelial lesion (HGSIL)** Here we see moderate to severe precancerous change, or "carcinoma in situ" (just shy of real cancer).

- **Invasive cancer**   This is the only classification term that is self-explanatory, and the last report we ever want to get. Thankfully, when women get regular Paps smears, it is rare.

Other terms you might need to know include:

- **Dysplasia** A term from an older classification system, dysplasia means precancer. It is graded as mild, moderate, or severe.

- **Cervical intraepithelial neoplasia (CIN)** This term is synonymous with dysplasia or precancer.

- **Microinvasive** Microinvasive is early cancer that has just barely broken into the surrounding tissues. It carries a better prognosis than frankly invasive cancer.

- **Colposcopy** A colposcopy is a detailed examination of the cervix and is explained in the next section.

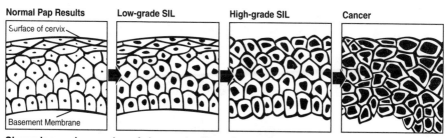

Shows increasing number of abnormal cells as the cervix progresses from normal to cancer.

Figure 7.2: Classification of cervical cells

What Is Done for a Patient with an Abnormal Pap Smear?

It is not uncommon for a woman to have an abnormal Pap smear at some time in her life. Cervical inflammation, precancer, and HPV infection are relatively common, and abnormal Paps are found in about 5 to 10% of samples. Also, Pap smears are a screening tool, which means they are meant to be super-sensitive in detecting precancer. In order to catch all precancer, the test will sometimes be too sensitive (i.e., the Pap is read as abnormal, but the cervix is really okay). The reverse also occurs, when the Pap fails to find precancer that actually exists; false negative Paps happen around 15% of the time (another good reason for women to have regular Paps).

When a woman has an abnormal Pap smear, she is often scheduled for an examination known as a colposcopy. During this exam, a gynecologist uses a colposcope (see Figure 7.3) to illuminate and magnify the cervix and look for evidence of

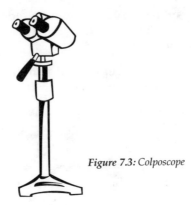

Figure 7.3: Colposcope

cancer or precancer. This procedure requires special training and practice. Colposcopy is performed as follows:

1. A speculum is placed in the vagina, just as is done for a Pap smear.
2. The cervix is cleaned with a diluted acetic acid (vinegar) solution.
3. A thorough visual exam is undertaken to look for evidence of precancer or cancer of the cervix. Abnormal areas are highlighted by the vinegar solution and the special filter on the colposcope. Precancerous tissue appears white and may have enlarged blood vessels on its surface.
4. Biopsies (tissue samples) are taken of any abnormal appearing areas. In addition, cells are often sampled from the canal of the cervix, because that area is difficult to evaluate visually.

Biopsies remove *tiny* fragments of tissue (about an eighth of an inch in size) and, thankfully, cause little if any pain for most patients. The cervix is far less sensitive than the vagina or the vulva, so local anesthesia is not necessary. Colposcopy takes between 15 and 30 minutes to complete, and most women have only slight discomfort afterward. The biopsies are sent to the pathologist for evaluation, and a report is made in a few days to a week.

What Is the Treatment for an Abnormal Cervix?

After the evaluation process is complete, the gynecologist interprets the biopsy findings to establish the final diagnosis.

Treatment is individualized and is based on the Pap smear, colposcopy findings, and biopsies (there should be agreement among these findings). Other factors may come into play, such as prior history of cervical or other genital disease, presence of other medical problems, and the likelihood of maintaining good follow-up with the patient. For the typical patient, the following approaches are often used:

- **Diagnosis: normal findings on biopsy/colposcopy** If the Pap was ASCUS or LGSIL, no treatment is needed. The doctor may repeat the Pap smear in six months to confirm that the cervix is free of disease.

  Note: If the Pap showed a high grade lesion, HGSIL, or cancer, and the colposcopy did *not* find disease, more investigation is often needed (see the sections on Cone biopsy and LEEP procedure, below).

- **Diagnosis: LGSIL, Human Papilloma Virus present** This is a very controversial area when it comes to treatment. Many physicians offer no treatment because studies have shown that if HPV is present on the cervix, it is probably also present throughout the genital tract: in the vagina, on the vulva, and around the rectum. Since no effective treatment can eradicate the virus from all areas, and no precancer has been found on biopsy, they see no reason to treat such a patient. Also, research has shown that in more than half of patients, this condition will resolve without treatment. Other physicians prefer to offer treatment because they have identified a focus of active viral replication that may progress to precancer and cancer if left alone. Treatment *may* also render the woman less infectious to her partner. Application of the same mild acid solution used on external warts has not been proven to decrease her chances of developing cancer later on, but it carries no significant risks. More aggressive treatments such as laser, cryotherapy, and surgery are generally not indicated for a woman with this diagnosis. At a minimum, Paps are repeated every six months for a year.

- **Diagnosis: LGSIL, mild dysplasia** When mild dysplasia, or precancer, is found on the external part of the cervix, most patients require no treatment, but are followed with Paps every six months for the next year. Most will regress on their own within one to two years.

One important exception: If the precancer extends into or lies within the cervical canal, the treatment approach is often to use Cone biopsy or the LEEP procedure (see below) to detect and remove any hidden disease.

- **Diagnosis: HGSIL, moderate or severe dysplasia** In the patient with this diagnosis, effective treatment is very important. Although 40% of HGSILs will regress spontaneously, a significant number of women, if left untreated, will develop cancer of the cervix. If the abnormal tissue can be seen in its entirety on the surface of the cervix, it can be treated with cryotherapy (freezing the outer cell layers of the cervix); 85% of patients are "cured" by this method. Cryotherapy is an office procedure and takes just a few minutes to complete. Patients experience moderate uterine cramping during the procedure, which rapidly resolves; some may have brief lightheadedness and flushing. A watery discharge is produced as the cervix thaws and begins to heal. The discharge lasts from ten to twenty days. We tell our patients to refrain from intercourse during this time, but any other activity (which doesn't involve the vagina) is okay.

If the precancerous tissue covers a large area of the cervix, or involves the cervical canal, a better approach may be to use minor surgery to remove it. The two ways we go about this are with Cone biopsy or the LEEP procedure. A Cone biopsy is exactly what it sounds like: using a knife or laser to remove a cone-shaped area of the cervix, which contains all the abnormal tissue. The Cone biopsy has been the "gold standard" approach to these patients for many years. It requires a brief visit to the operating room, and usually the patient can return home the same day. However, the side effects of this minor surgery can be substantial; they include heavy bleeding (rarely, transfusion may be necessary), infection, and damage to the cervix. A woman who has had a Cone biopsy may even have difficulty carrying a pregnancy to term because the cervix has been weakened.

LEEP stands for loop electrosurgical excision procedure. In this treatment approach, a tiny electrified wire loop is passed around the precancerous portion of the cervix, thereby removing it. LEEPs can usually be done in the office. They are quicker, less costly, and have fewer side effects than Cone biopsies. LEEPs may be replacing the Cone biopsy as the treatment of choice because of these differences. Whether a Cone biopsy or LEEP procedure is used, the removed tissue needs careful analysis by a pathologist. Unless cancer is found, the patient is followed with Pap smears every six months for two to three years. As with mild precancer, if any of the following Paps are abnormal, colposcopy will often again be necessary.

- **Diagnosis: "carcinoma in situ" (CIS)** The standard approach to a patient with CIS is a Cone biopsy. Even with this treatment, there is a chance the disease will persist (6%) or progress to cancer (0.6%). Long-term follow-up with Pap smears and colposcopy is especially crucial in women diagnosed with CIS. In the past, many gynecologists performed a hysterectomy (removal of the uterus) for CIS, believing the risks of progression to cancer might be too high. Current data from studies do not bear this out. However, a woman with any other indication for hysterectomy would be advised to have that surgery if she also has CIS.

- **Diagnosis: cervical cancer** Thankfully, cervical cancer is a rare result of the investigation of an abnormal Pap smear in women who have regular care. Treatment options for cervical cancer are beyond the scope of this book but include standard and "radical" hysterectomy and radiation therapy. Gynecologists with special surgical and medical training in cancer treatment, gynecologic oncologists, provide excellent care for these patients.

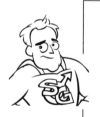

Tips for Supportive Guys If Their Partner Has an Abnormal Pap Smear

Now that you know all about abnormal pap smears, what are you going to do about it? Some suggestions:

1. Find out what her diagnosis is. Then use the information presented here to help her understand the planned treatment. If she's not sure about her diagnosis, encourage her to find out (you can call her doctor also).

(continued)

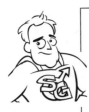

2. Be supportive of her emotional state. It is understandably frightening for her to have an abnormal Pap smear. If she happens to cry, try just letting her without trying to stop it. Hugs are good at times like this.

   Most importantly, listen to what she has to say. According to noted male-female communication expert Pat Heim, Ph.D., men should let go of the urge to "fix" their partners' problems and instead simply ask questions and listen. Try asking, "How did that make you feel to go through that?" and "What's the next step?" as well as the biggie: "What can I do to help you with this?" This approach will work better, and you'll both be happier.

3. Be patient if she needs time to heal after colposcopy or treatment. She may not be able to make love for a little while, but she'll probably *need* love.

4. Offer to accompany her to the doctor. Many women have told us how much they appreciate this gesture. They feel this way even if their partners don't understand much about their problem.

5. If she smokes, encourage her to quit. She probably already knows that lung cancer kills more women than breast cancer. She may not know smoking increases her risks of bladder, throat, and cervical cancer. If you smoke, try inspiring by example (quit!).

6. Be reassuring. Abnormal Paps are common—cervical cancer is not. Major surgery (i.e., hysterectomy) is rarely necessary.

7. Encourage her to have all the appropriate treatment and follow-up recommended by her doctor. Remind her that precancer, which is treatable, causes no symptoms—only advanced cancer of the cervix does. Close follow-up is usually necessary for two to three years, and then annual Paps are needed for life. Don't let down your support.

ENDOMETRIOSIS

What Is Endometriosis?

Simply stated, endometriosis is the presence of endometrial (uterine lining) tissue outside of the uterine cavity, usually in the pelvis. This can be a very severe, debilitating disease. Although not life-threatening, it has the following nasty habits:

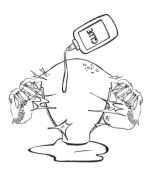

- Endometriosis can act like cancer and invade other tissues.

- Endometriosis often causes scarring (called adhesions) within the pelvis, binding structures together and distorting anatomy. This may lead to chronic pain and infertility.

- Endometriosis may occur in cystic collections, called endometriomas, on the ovaries. These can reach several inches in diameter and can cause severe pain, requiring urgent surgical removal.

A woman with endometriosis may suffer for many years with all of these problems. Interestingly, some women with extensive disease have few or no symptoms. Because of its unpredictability and potential severity, endometriosis is one of the most challenging illnesses gynecologists face.

Why Does Endometriosis Cause These Problems?

Recall from Chapter 1 (see "Female Anatomy" and "The Menstrual Cycle") that the endometrium is the inner lining of the uterus. The endometrium thickens and matures during each menstrual cycle in response to estrogen and progesterone, readying the uterus for pregnancy. When a pregnancy fails to occur, this lining tissue sloughs and bleeds (this is a woman's period, or menses). If there is endometrial tissue *outside* the uterus as well, this same cell proliferation (thickening), sloughing, and bleeding can lead to all the problems described in the previous section.

Endometriosis is common! It has been found in 8 to 30% of women undergoing pelvic surgeries. We see the disease most commonly in women in their 20s and 30s, but it can occur in patients in their teen years to those in the menopause. It seems to have a hereditary component, often occurring in women of the same family over several generations.

What Causes Endometriosis?

The two most common theories on the causes of endometriosis are transportation of endometrial tissue out of the uterine cavity and transformation of other tissues into an endometrial type. The transportation theory suggests that endometrial tissue may escape from the uterus and implant in other areas of the body. We know that women with a narrow or blocked cervical opening may have endometrial tissue flow out of the fallopian tubes during their periods because it can't leave the normal way. Endometriosis has also been found at sites distant from the pelvis, such as the lungs, an arm or leg, or in surgical scars. This suggests that endometrial tissue was transported either by the circulatory system or directly during surgery, and was able to implant and grow.

The transformation theory, called coelomic metaplasia, explains the presence of pelvic endometriosis by suggesting that certain primitive cells within the pelvic cavity have the capacity to mature to an endometrial cell type, given the proper hormonal stimulation.

Current wisdom says that both the transportation and transformation theories have merit and may be operable to varying degrees in each patient with the disease. Some researchers believe that a woman with endometriosis may be predisposed to the disease because she has a biochemical defect that allows or promotes it.

What Symptoms Does Endometriosis Cause?

A woman with endometriosis may have mild, vague pelvic pain, moderate symptoms, or she may be completely debilitated. She may have microscopic endometrial implants that are invisible to the naked eye, or the entire pelvis, including the uterus, tubes, ovaries, and bowel may be matted down with adhesions and distorted beyond recognition. *The symptoms often do not coincide with the extent of the disease.* The location of the endometriosis within the pelvis, rather than how much there is or how long it's been there, seems to be most important in terms of causing pain. In addition to pelvic pain, the most common symptoms of endometriosis are infertility and abnormal bleeding.

Pelvic pain from endometriosis can take one or more forms. A woman may have intermittent, spontaneous pain unrelated to her menstrual cycle, ranging from mild to severe. It may be experienced as a dull lower backache, sharp pelvic pains, or rectal or lower pelvic pressure, depending on the location of the endometrial implants. The woman may also have painful periods, with menstrual cramps, rectal pressure, bowel irritability, or radiating pains into the vagina or the thighs.

Does it *really* hurt? One gynecologist in Washington tells the partners of his endometriosis patients to "imagine having one of your *testicles* taped tightly to your thigh and running around all day."

Pain with intercourse may develop, especially if the endometriosis involves the cul-de-sac beneath the uterus (during sex, this area gets a lot of contact). In addition, endometriosis may cause one or both ovaries to become bound tightly to the uterus, which increases their sensitivity.

Pain with bowel movements may occur if the disease has invaded the bowels or caused adhesions between the bowel and other organs within the pelvis.

Infertility is a frequent problem in patients with endometriosis. Estimates state that 30 to 40% of infertile women have some degree of endometriosis, although it may not be causing their infertility. When extensive scar tissue from endometriosis involving the ovaries and tubes is found during surgery, the cause of the infertility is clear. Interestingly, many women with mild endometriosis and no visible anatomic distortion may also have problems getting pregnant. This may be caused by the local effects of chemicals produced by the displaced endometrial tissue.

Abnormal bleeding occurs in up to one-third of patients with endometriosis. Menstrual periods may become irregular, prolonged, or heavier than normal; light menstrual spotting may be seen for days before the flow begins. The bleeding changes are not completely understood but may be caused by chemicals produced by the abnormal endometrial tissue.

Other symptoms seen with endometriosis are less common but can occur when the disease implants in and/or invades unusual locations. These symptoms include rectal bleeding, bladder pain, bloody urine, cough, chest pain, bloody sputum, and pain in surgical scars.

How Is Endometriosis Diagnosed?

The classic findings of endometriosis that can be discovered during a physical exam are a result of implantation of endometrial tissue in the space between the uterus and the rectum: tenderness and irregularity of the cul-de-sac and the utero-sacral ligaments. In addition, an enlarged and tender ovary may be detected in a patient with an endometrioma (a cystic collection of endometriosis and blood on an ovary).

An enlarged ovary with an endometrioma may also be detected with an ultrasound examination. This provides helpful information in a patient with other findings suggestive of endometriosis, but it isn't specific enough to make a definite diagnosis. Sometimes the ultrasound exam discloses *another* cause for the patient's symptoms, such as an ovarian cyst or fibroid tumors of the uterus. There are no good blood tests for endometriosis at present. Before too long, however, researchers may find a specific chemical marker for the disease that can be measured easily in the blood.

Endometriosis can only be definitively diagnosed at surgery; no combination of symptoms and physical findings provides complete certainty without confirmation with either laparoscopy or open surgery (laparotomy). Many women who don't have endometriosis have painful periods or pelvic pain. We stress the need for visual and/or biopsy-proven diagnosis because we have treated women who were "diagnosed" with endometriosis without surgery who probably never had the disease. The psychological and physical impact of the misdiagnosis of endometriosis can be severe, making this a crucial issue for women.

How Is Endometriosis Treated?

Treatment for the woman with endometriosis is often difficult. There are many different approaches, and the treatment plan should be individualized, based on the severity, location, and extent of the disease, as well as the woman's wishes with regard to fertility and surgery. Having endometriosis does not mean she will have to have a hysterectomy. Treatment alternatives range from observation and pain relievers to the use of medical suppression (drug treatment) and minor or major surgery.

Observation (no treatment) may be chosen for women with mild disease and few symptoms. Often these patients have had a recent diagnosis made at laparoscopy at which time the disease was treated with cautery, laser vaporization, or excision (removal) of the involved tissue. Since some endometrial implants and scar tissue may remain after surgery, this cannot be counted on to produce a cure. Nonnarcotic pain medications such as ibuprofen may be all that is needed, and the disease may regress on its own.

For women with endometriosis whose primary complaint is pain, but who might want to have children in the future, the first step is usually conservative surgery. Conservative surgery, as used here, means removal of only the endometrial implants and the adhesions they have caused. No pelvic organs are removed or interfered with, if possible. The intention is to relieve pain and restore normal anatomy while not interfering with future fertility. Occasionally the disease is severe enough to require removal of an ovary and/or a fallopian tube in order to relieve the patient's pain, but every attempt is made to leave everything in place and ready for pregnancy.

Conservative surgery may be performed through a standard abdominal incision or, as is increasingly popular, via laparoscopy. Laparoscopy uses long, narrow instruments and a fiber-optic scope placed through two to four tiny (one quarter to half an inch) abdominal incisions to visualize and operate in the pelvis. High-resolution video cameras allow surgeons to watch the operation on a closed-circuit TV screen as they perform it. More information on laparoscopy, and other gynecologic surgery techniques, can be found in Chapter 8.

After conservative surgery, medications are often given to further suppress the disease. Treatments that create either a low-estrogen state (endometrial tissue is highly dependent on estrogen stimulation) or a high-progesterone state like pregnancy seem to be helpful in suppressing endometriosis.

Taking birth control pills creates a hormonal environment similar to pregnancy. To gain their full effect on the endometriosis, it takes six to nine months; therefore, this approach is not popular with patients in significant pain. Progesterone may be used by itself in oral or injectable form, but this may have bothersome side effects, such as irregular periods or depression.

A potent way to lower estrogen levels is found with a new class of medicines called the Gn RH agonists. These drugs cause a profound fall in estrogen levels by stopping the brain's stimulation of the ovaries. Side effects include hot flashes, vaginal dryness, insomnia, and mood swings, but relief of pain is substantial in most patients after one to two months. Therapy cannot be continued for more than six months with the Gn RH agonists, because the low-estrogen state leads to bone loss. Studies are underway on the effects of giving a small amount of estrogen and/or progesterone during Gn RH therapy (so-called "add-back" therapy) to prevent bone loss, decrease side effects, and allow longer treatment.

Additional research has begun on the effectiveness of RU-486, the much-maligned French abortion pill, in treating endometriosis. Preliminary results are encouraging.

For women with endometriosis whose primary concern is infertility, conservative surgery alone seems to be the favored approach. As mentioned above, conservative surgery is usually done through the laparoscope. Only the endometriosis is removed (along with any scarring that has resulted), and the pelvic organs are left intact whenever possible. If a woman wishes to become pregnant immediately, it's usually best to avoid using hormonal medications like birth control pills, progesterone, or the Gn RH agonists after surgery.

Pregnancy rates following conservative surgery for endometriosis range from 30 to 94%, based on how much endometriosis existed before the operation. In studies to date, many will conceive by six months and most within two years.

Finally, for women with endometriosis who either have severe pain that is unresponsive to other treatments or who don't want children, more aggressive surgery is often the best answer. This more "radical" surgical approach is an attempt to cure the disease once and for all by removing all visible endometriosis as well as the source of estrogen production that stimulates it, the ovaries. Usually the uterus and tubes are removed as well, especially if they are also involved with the disease. If there is a normal ovary without evidence of disease, it may be left with only a small chance of recurrence of endometriosis. If both ovaries are removed, estrogen levels fall permanently. Most of these women are candidates for low-dose estrogen replacement, which usually does not cause the disease to recur.

Women with endometriosis are best served with early diagnosis, education, effective treatment, and close follow-up. The disease varies in its course and is often difficult to manage, both for a woman and her physician. As her partner, you are sure to be affected by the endometriosis as well.

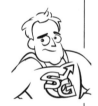

What Can I Do If My Partner Has Endometriosis?

How you react is important; here are some suggestions:

- Be patient and understanding. She has an unpredictable and often painful disease affecting her reproductive organs, which may require surgery. Imagine how you'd feel (recall the testicle-taped-to-the-thigh analogy).

- Be a good listener. Remember, women deal with emotion by processing, not just talking. Ask questions like "What happens next?" "How are you feeling about this?" "What can I do to help?" Then, just listen and don't try to "fix" her.

- Be gentle with her during intercourse. She may have moderate or severe pain during or afterward. Be open to variations in position. Certain times of the month (typically, midcycle and during her period) may be more painful for her.

(continued)

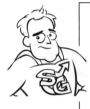

- Encourage doctor visits for follow-up, especially if she's having trouble with pain or irregular periods. Early treatment is often simpler and more effective.
- Go with her to the doctor's office, or talk to her doctor by phone. If you've taken the time to educate yourself (by reading this book, for example), your questions should be well received. Her endometriosis affects both of you, and she'll appreciate your interest.
- Do something nice for her. Make sure she understands you'll hang in there with her through this difficult time.

UTERINE FIBROIDS

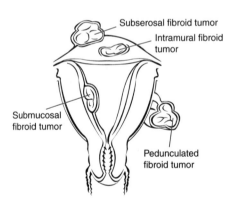

Subserosal fibroid tumor

Intramural fibroid tumor

Submucosal fibroid tumor

Pedunculated fibroid tumor

Uterine fibroids, also known as leiomyomata uteri or myomas, are the most common tumor of the uterus and the female pelvis. Twenty percent of reproductive-age females have them, and the percentage increases as age increases. Fibroids are more common in African American women and are often found in several women in the same family. Fibroids are the most common reason for pelvic surgery in women, accounting for nearly one-third of hysterectomies for noncancers.

What Are Uterine Fibroids?

Each tumor starts from a single muscle cell within the uterus. It may be tiny, detectable only with a microscope, or it may grow as large as 100 pounds. A woman may have a single fibroid or several dozen. They may grow within the wall of the uterus (called intramural myomas), into the endometrial cavity (submucosal myomas), or extend from the uterus into the pelvic cavity (subserosal or pedunculated).

The growth of fibroids appears to be dependent on estrogen. High-estrogen states like pregnancy usually stimulate fibroid growth, and low-estrogen states like the menopause will often cause the tumors to shrink. Modern low-dose oral contraceptives do *not* cause fibroid growth.

What Symptoms Do They Cause?

The symptoms produced by fibroids are a function of their size, number, and location within the uterus. Most women with small fibroids have few if any complaints and require no treatment.

The most common symptom, however, is heavy menstrual bleeding, seen in one-third of women with fibroids. The increased bleeding may be caused by changes in blood flow within the uterus or abnormal blood vessels in the fibroid itself. Iron-deficiency anemia (a low red blood cell count) is a frequent finding in women with heavy bleeding caused by fibroids.

Pelvic pain, pressure, discomfort with sex, irregular bleeding, and cramps also are often mentioned as symptoms. Less commonly, urinary frequency (from compression of the bladder), constipation (from pressure on the colon), and infertility may result from fibroids. Severe pain may result from degeneration of a fibroid tumor if it outgrows its blood supply.

Pregnant women with fibroids usually give birth to normal infants but have a slightly higher risk of a number of complications. Miscarriages, premature labor, pelvic pain, abnormal presentation of the fetus (not headfirst), rupture of the uterus, premature separation of the placenta, and postdelivery hemorrhage are seen more often in these pregnancies. Cesarean section is also more common in the pregnancy complicated with fibroids. More frequent prenatal visits and special precautions may be necessary in these pregnancies.

How Are Uterine Fibroids Diagnosed?

The diagnosis of fibroids is relatively simple. If the fibroids are large, a pelvic exam usually will discover them. A sonogram or pelvic ultrasound may be helpful to distinguish a fibroid uterus from a solid ovarian tumor or other pelvic mass. The diagnosis of a submucosal fibroid (within the endometrial cavity) may be made by hysteroscopy—the use of a tiny fiber-optic scope placed through the cervix. This approach compliments the D & C, a "blind" procedure that has been shown to miss many polyps and fibroids. A sonogram may sometimes diagnose a submucosal fibroid as well.

 D & C means *dilation* of the cervix and *curettage* or scraping of the uterine lining. Dilation of the cervix is necessary to accommodate the scraping instrument, since the cervix is ordinarily almost closed. The procedure usually takes 5 or 10 minutes to complete, and recovery is quick. Chapter 8, which covers gynecologic surgery, will describe the alternatives to D & C. The newer procedures (such as hysteroscopy) are often simpler and safer and obtain more information than a standard D & C.

Complications from fibroids that may require surgery include sudden hemorrhage (bleeding), degeneration with severe pain, and cancerous change (one in 200 patients). Rapid growth of the uterus over a period of a few months is suggestive of a cancer.

How Are Uterine Fibroids Treated?

The management of a patient with uterine fibroids has changed in the past few years. No longer do we see as many hysterectomies done simply because of the presence of a moderately enlarged uterus (the so-called "Because it's there!" approach). The goal should be to use all available medical and minor surgical options to manage the patient's symptoms, resorting to hysterectomy only as a last resort. The approach must be individualized, based on each patient's overall health, the effect of her fibroids on adjacent organs, and her wishes with regard to fertility.

The traditional approach to a patient with symptomatic uterine fibroids has been an abdominal or vaginal hysterectomy. This is still a very good choice for many patients who have no desire for future pregnancy and do not wish to accept the alternative forms of treatment. Two other surgical choices are hysteroscopy with removal of submucosal myomas (fibroids within the uterine cavity) and myomectomy.

Hysteroscopy with removal of submucosal myomas appears to be safe and effective in treating bleeding problems caused by small or moderately sized tumors in the uterus. This operation uses a highly specialized fiber-optic scope placed within the uterus to locate and remove the tumors. A secondary procedure called endometrial ablation actually removes most or all of the lining of the uterus to further decrease bleeding. Both of these are outpatient operations (patients go home the same day).

Myomectomy is a popular treatment choice for those patients who wish to preserve their uterus for future childbearing or other reasons. This operation involves removing all the fibroids from the body of the uterus. This can be a difficult procedure, sometimes resulting in an emergency hysterectomy because of uncontrolled bleeding. Blood transfusions are given more commonly for myomectomy (10–15%) than for hysterectomy (5–10%). Scar tissue may form after this type of surgery, causing infertility or blockage of the intestines. If many fibroids were removed or if the uterine cavity was entered during the surgery, the patient may require cesarean section with future pregnancies. Sometimes the myomas can be removed through a laparoscope and three or four small (half inch) incisions. This requires a highly trained surgeon.

Fibroids often recur after these operations. Any patient having either hysteroscopic removal of a myoma or myomectomy should be aware that there is at least a 20% chance that she will need future surgery for the same condition at some time.

The medical approach to the treatment of uterine fibroids uses a medicine that causes estrogen levels to fall. Gn RH agonists are a new class of medicines that do this by stopping the pituitary's stimulation of the ovaries. The drugs are given as intramuscular injections or are inhaled through the nose. Shrinkage of myomas is seen in about two months, with a maximum effect by three to six months. The medicines are usually not taken beyond six months because the lowered estrogen levels in the body cause osteopenia (loss of bone). Unfortunately, once the medication is stopped, the fibroids will usually regrow within six to twelve months.

Current research is focused on the effect of giving a small amount of estrogen or progesterone along with the Gn RH agonist, to protect the bones. If this research is successful, treatment could be prolonged in some patients.

The side effects of Gn RH agonists are a result of the low levels of estrogen in the body. Hot flashes, vaginal dryness, insomnia, painful intercourse, and mood swings, typical of menopause, are often reported. Irregular bleeding may occur as well, but more often menstrual flow stops altogether after a month of therapy.

The overall size of the uterus may decrease by up to 60% during treatment with Gn RH agonists. This initial shrinkage reduces many of the symptoms caused by the tumors and also may allow a woman to have a vaginal rather than an abdominal hysterectomy (which usually means a shorter and easier recovery).

Pre-operative anemia (low blood count) can be rapidly treated with iron supplements because Gn RH agonists usually stop heavy menstrual bleeding. This is important because women are less likely to need a blood transfusion after hysterectomy if their red blood cell count is normal before the operation.

In addition, the Gn RH agonists along with other medications may allow some women to avoid hysterectomy if they are nearing menopause. Typically, bleeding problems diminish in severity with the onset of the menopause.

 A new medicine currently being investigated for the treatment of myomas is RU-486, the French abortion pill. Recent studies of this anti-progesterone compound at the University of California at San Diego showed a 49% reduction in fibroid volume after three months. Preliminary reports are positive, with 9 of 10 patients responding well to the treatment.

A. A. Murphy et al., *Fertility and Sterility* 64(1): 187–90 (1995).

Fibroid tumors of the uterus are truly a common problem. Many women with fibroids have few if any symptoms and can be treated without surgery. The chance that the tumors will become malignant (cancerous) is less than one percent. If the fibroids cause heavy bleeding or pain because of their size or location, surgery of various types may be an excellent choice. New medications like the Gn RH agonists may be able to "buy time" to improve a low blood count and/or allow a vaginal hysterectomy. With advancing knowledge, use of these medicines may allow some women to avoid surgery altogether.

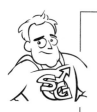

What You Can Do If Your Partner Has Fibroids

- Reassure her that major surgery isn't often needed and that cancerous fibroids are very rare.

- Reinforce the need for follow-up with her doctor at regular intervals. If she's pregnant, urge her to get close follow-up with an obstetrician or a perinatologist (a specialist in high-risk pregnancies).

- Discuss the plan for managing the fibroids with her. Help her remember her medications (if necessary).

- Be gentle with intercourse, as she may have pelvic pain caused by the fibroids.

- If she needs an operation (either major or minor), go with her to the hospital. Make sure you understand what happened in surgery and the plan for follow-up (for more information on surgery, see Chapter 8).

- As always, ask her how she's feeling both physically and emotionally. Be a good listener.

POST TEST

1. One reason women have more bladder infections than men is because they have a shorter urethra.

   T or F

2. Vitamin E taken after intercourse reduces the frequency of bladder infections.

   T or F

3. A mammogram is the only way to diagnose a breast cancer.

   T or F

4. Most breast lumps are found *not* to be cancerous.

   T or F

5. The Human Papilloma Virus is responsible for the majority of abnormal Pap smears in young women today.

   T or F

6. Cervical cancer is much more common in countries where Pap smears aren't done.

   T or F

7. Penicillin is the drug of choice to cure endometriosis.

   T or F

8. Infertility is a potential problem for women with endometriosis.

   T or F

9. Fibroid tumors in the uterus are often cancerous and must be removed immediately when diagnosed.

   T or F

10. Heavy periods and pelvic pain are often the result of fibroids.

    T or F

Key: 1. T   2. F   3. F   4. T   5. T   6. T   7. F   8. T   9. F   10. T

UNDER THE KNIFE: GYNECOLOGIC SURGERY

8

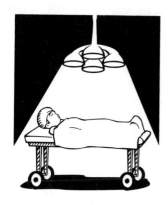

Too few blankets on your barely covered body. No familiar faces. Waiting. Waiting more. People rushing around, looking at you but not speaking. Finally, questions: "Are you allergic to anything?"

"Have you ever had surgery before?" "What medicines do you take?" The same questions repeated by someone else five minutes later. Waiting again. Thirsty.

(Where's my doctor?)

Being rolled down a long sterile corridor on a gurney. Strange sounds, loud noises. People talking with words you don't understand. A masked person says, "Don't worry . . . everything will be fine."

(What if something goes wrong?)

In the operating room: stark, white, very cold. Huge lights hanging from the ceiling. Trays, tables, lots of "things," big machines with lights and dials. Being rolled or lifted onto a hard flat table in the center of it all. Looking up into those big lights, surrounded by all those machines.

(Why do I feel so exposed?)

Wires stuck to your chest, your stomach, your hands. An IV carries some unknown fluid directly into your bloodstream. Arms "positioned," legs "positioned." Above your head, that masked person you don't know says, "Everything will be fine. You're going off to sleep now."

(I can't move . . . !)

We all have some version of these thoughts when we surrender our bodies to a surgeon. Whether the operation is minor or major, fear finds us all at some point in the process.

And it's normal to be afraid before surgery! To undergo an operation is to surrender your control of the only body you'll ever have. As we will detail in this chapter, every procedure carries risks: there is the chance of dangerous blood loss or infection; anesthesia can be hazardous; organs can be permanently damaged during an operation.

The good news is that the vast majority of gynecologic operations are accomplished without complication and produce excellent results. We, your doctors, are rigorously trained to bring you safely through surgery. This is a sacred trust. To be allowed to open a person's body in order to help her is perhaps the greatest honor of being a physician.

Much of what happens in the O.R., however, is a mystery to most nonmedical people. Patients and their families have typically learned a little about a planned procedure only because they were imminently faced with it, but that's a difficult time to really understand something so frightening and important.

Thankfully times are changing. Medical shows on television make a better attempt to simulate reality; some cable channels regularly feature real, live operations! The internet is already loaded with information on surgeries of many kinds, as well as alternative forms of treatment. What's driving this change is that, now, people want to know before the last minute. We applaud this change.

Your reading of this book is an example of that search for information. Now that you have learned the basics about women's health, it's time to learn a little about the surgeries we do. As always, this knowledge will make you a better partner.

In this chapter, we will present useful and somewhat detailed information on four of the more common gynecologic surgeries. We will introduce you to the **D & C**, a useful minor operation. Next, we cover surgery for **ovarian cysts** and **ectopic pregnancies**. The chapter concludes by covering the **hysterectomy**, a major operation done commonly by gynecologists.

For each of these operations, we answer: Why does she need the operation? What are the alternative treatments? What are the risks of surgery? This information should help both of you understand her planned treatment. It may even prompt a discussion with her doctor about delaying surgery or adopting another treatment plan altogether.

This chapter includes subsections ("What Happens During the Surgery?") that describe many of the steps doctors go through to safely complete each operation. You may find this information makes you uneasy, and then again it may fascinate you. Skip over these subsections if you'd like.

At the end of the chapter, we answer: What can I do to help? If you read nothing else, don't miss this. Your participation at this frightening time, both before and after surgery, can make your partner feel significantly better.

GUY-Q TEST

1. Surgical risks include:
   a. blood loss requiring transfusion.
   b. developing an infection at the site of the operation.
   c. anesthesia complications.
   d. damage to structures surrounding the site of the operation.
   e. all of the above.

2. A D & C is:
   a. sterilization surgery.
   b. treatment for infection of the cervix.
   c. dilation of the cervix and curettage (scraping) of the uterine lining.

3. A D & C might be used to treat:
   a. persistent abnormal bleeding from the uterus.
   b. a miscarriage.
   c. a lost IUD.
   d. all of the above.

4. Ovarian cysts may:
   a. rupture, causing severe pain.
   b. bleed into the abdomen, causing shock.
   c. grow to very large sizes.
   d. all of the above.

5. Abnormal bleeding from the uterus can often be controlled by:
   a. birth control pills.
   b. progesterone injections.
   c. correction of thyroid deficiency.
   d. all of the above.

6. An ectopic pregnancy is:
   a. a pregnancy inside the uterus that is not growing normally.
   b. a pregnancy that is growing outside the uterus.
   c. a pregnancy that is compromised by drugs or alcohol.

7. Ectopic pregnancies:
   a. comprise one to two percent of all pregnancies.
   b. can be placed in the uterus if detected early enough.
   c. can cause death from internal bleeding if not treated in time.
   d. can lead to infertility if the fallopian tubes are damaged.
   e. all but b.

8. Treatments for ectopic pregnancy include:
   a. surgery on the involved segment of fallopian tube.
   b. medical therapy with an anticancer drug, methotrexate.
   c. in selected cases, careful observation only.
   d. all of the above.

9. A total hysterectomy indicates removal of:
   a. the uterus and cervix.
   b. the uterus, cervix, tubes, and ovaries.
   c. the uterus, cervix, and appendix.

10. Indications for hysterectomy may include:
    a. large, growing fibroid tumors of the uterus.
    b. uncontrollable uterine bleeding.
    c. cancer of the uterus, cervix, or ovaries.
    d. loss of pelvic support leading to the dropping of the uterus into the vagina.
    e. all of the above.

Key: 1. e   2. c   3. d   4. d   5. d   6. b   7. e   8. d   9. a   10. e

D & C

A D & C is known among lay persons as a "dusting and cleaning" of the uterus, or, in medical parlance, "dilation and curettage." In the operating room, the cervix is opened (dilation) and the superficial lining of the uterus (the endometrium) is removed (curettage). It is a low-tech procedure, usually requiring only minutes to complete. One of the oldest surgeries in use today, the D & C is often replaced or improved by newer medical and surgical techniques.

Over its long history, the D & C has been used to treat many different problems. At the present time, it is used most commonly to treat abnormal uterine bleeding that has not responded to medications. Women experiencing a prolonged and heavy menstrual flow may have a D & C to stop their blood loss. Women who suffer from a condition known as dysfunctional uterine bleeding, which is characterized by persistent irregular bleeding, may also have a D & C (for more on this condition, see the addendum at the end of this section). The D & C can be used to detect and remove polyps or fibroids within the cavity of the uterus; however, hysteroscopy is probably better (discussed below in the section on alternatives).

Another common use for the D & C is to remove a nonliving early pregnancy from the uterus. Between 15 and 20% of pregnancies detected by standard pregnancy tests result in a nonsurviving embryo. Terms applied to this condition include missed abortion, spontaneous abortion, miscarriage, and blighted ovum. Without a D & C, most women would have prolonged, painful cramping and bleeding as the uterus expels the pregnancy on its own. It is standard practice to evacuate the uterus with a D & C once we know the embryo is not living.

Irregular bleeding, especially in a postmenopausal woman, may signal cancer of the uterus. A biopsy of the uterus (endometrial biopsy) done in the office can exclude this diagnosis in most cases. If the office biopsy cannot be done for any reason or if the results are inconclusive, a woman may need a D & C.

Finally, a D & C may be needed to remove a lost IUD. As discussed in Chapter 2, intrauterine devices have a string on one end that hangs out of the cervix. Feeling the string allows a woman to verify that the IUD is in place and working. If the string cannot be found, it is usually necessary to locate and remove the IUD. Usually this can be accomplished in the office, but occasionally a D & C is performed.

What Are the Alternatives to a D & C?

Alternative treatments for D & C could fill a chapter all by themselves. A few examples:

- For heavy uterine bleeding: Heavy bleeding can some-times be stopped with oral or intravenous high-dose hormone treatment. Estrogen and/or progesterone can be used to stabilize the endometrium (e.g., high-dose birth control pills).

- For irregular uterine bleeding: Bleeding between menstrual periods is often caused by fibroids or polyps within the uterine cavity. Recent studies have suggested that it is easier to find and treat these problems with hysteroscopy than with D & C alone.

  As mentioned in Chapter 7, hysteroscopy is performed with a long, narrow fiber-optic scope. The scope is placed through the cervix so the doctor can view the uterine cavity. Specialized instruments can then be used to remove any abnormalities. A surgeon performing a D & C will often miss these same lesions because he or she cannot see inside the uterus.

One study evaluated 29 patients with persistent abnormal bleeding. When D & C was used to evaluate them, only one patient was found to have a fibroid causing her bleeding. Hysteroscopy was then used, and 19 of the 29 were found to have fibroids!

P. G. Brooks et al., "Hysteroscopic findings after unsuccessful dilation and curettage for abnormal uterine bleeding," *American Journal of Obstetrics and Gynecology* 158(6, part 1): 1354–7 (1988).

- For a nonsurviving embryo: Nonsurviving embryos in early pregnancy are most often treated with a D & C. On some occasions, all of the pregnancy has been passed by the time a woman is examined. In this circumstance, if the bleeding is minimal and there are no signs of infection, no treatment may be required. If the pregnancy has grown beyond 12 weeks before expiring, it is usually removed by prostaglandin induction of labor instead of by D & C. Prostaglandins are powerful hormones that stimulate uterine contractions and facilitate emptying of the uterus.

- For a "lost" IUD: A lost IUD can often be retrieved in the office with specialized instruments. When this isn't successful, hysteroscopy has become the preferred procedure to find and remove the IUD.

- To rule out uterine cancer as the cause of abnormal bleeding: Measurement of the thickness of the uterine lining with a sonogram may be used to exclude the diagnosis of uterine cancer. A very thin uterine lining is unlikely to be cancerous.

What Are the Risks of a D & C?

Surgery of any kind is not without significant risk, and all patients should be informed in advance of those risks whenever possible. Informed Consent is obtained from every patient before surgery, and all risks, benefits, and alternatives of the planned procedure are reviewed. Thorough documentation of this conversation is placed in the chart.

Of course, it's also possible to go too far with informed consent. When a simple and straightforward surgery is planned, too detailed a presentation about all possible risks can be unnecessarily frightening. Risk is a part of surgery, but with a competent surgeon, serious complications are very rare. A balanced presentation that enables a person to make an informed decision about his or her treatment is the ultimate goal.

Four basic risks apply to all operations:

- **Infection** Surgery involves the introduction of instruments into the body and temporarily disrupts normal anatomy. The tissue damage that occurs increases the risk of infection. Antibiotics and/or local treatment (cleaning the wound) may be needed if infection occurs.

- **Bleeding** Depending on the patient, the type of surgery, and the skill of the surgeon, significant blood loss may occur. The body can usually tolerate blood loss of more than a unit (500cc) without complication. Replacement of lost blood with intravenous fluids or blood (transfusion) may be necessary. Patients are informed of the opportunity to donate their own blood in advance, if so desired.

Blood from the blood bank (donor blood from the community) undergoes an extensive battery of tests before it is released for use. Tests are performed for various types of infection, including hepatitis and HIV. Current estimates put the risk of acquiring serious disease at well below one percent per unit transfused.

- **Anesthesia**   Various types of anesthesia are available for patients during surgery, from local to "regional" (e.g., spinal) to general. Risk occurs with anesthesia because of the effects of the very potent medicines used. The risks are compounded when patients come to surgery as an emergency, and/or with complicated medical conditions. Problems range from a headache after spinal anesthesia to death from complications from general anesthesia. Well-trained anethesiologists do an amazing job of keeping patients safe and comfortable during and after their operation.

- **Injury to surrounding structures**   A D & C for instance carries the risk of perforation of the uterus. If a perforation occurs, the intestines or bladder (which are nearby) could be damaged. If this happens, laparoscopy or open surgery may be needed to repair the injuries. Each type of surgery carries similar risk to the body part being operated on, and all surrounding structures.

What Happens During the Surgery?

After arrival in the O.R., the patient is positioned on the operating table appropriately for the planned operation. If it hasn't been done, an IV is started and fluids are given. Monitors are placed on the patient to follow blood pressure, heart rate and oxygen saturation in the blood. A mask with oxygen is placed on or near the patient's mouth.

If a general anesthetic is to be used, the anesthesiologist gives medications through the IV to slowly induce sleep and muscle relaxation. Once the patient is fully asleep, a breathing tube may be placed in the trachea (windpipe). The nurses prepare the surgical site by washing it thoroughly and shaving it where necessary. Sterile drapes are placed around the area. A catheter may be inserted into the bladder opening to keep the bladder empty during the operation. Draining the bladder helps to protect it from injury.

All operating personnel wear sterile gowns and gloves along with protective eyewear, hair covers, and masks. Universal precautions, which mandate separation of the operating team from all body fluids of the patient (and vice versa), are followed. This practice, inspired by the HIV epidemic, protects both the operating team and the patient during surgery.

For a D & C, the following steps are taken next: The medical team places her feet in stirrups. The vagina is cleaned with mild soap. The cervix is dilated a small amount to allow the passage of a curette. This instrument gently removes the superficial lining of the uterine cavity. Any tissue obtained is sent to the pathologist for microscopic examination.

If the D & C is for a nonliving pregnancy, a small suction catheter may be used in addition to the curette to speed the evacuation of the uterus. If an IUD is to be removed, other instruments may be used to grasp it.

The procedure is terminated by checking for excessive bleeding, and then carefully removing all instruments. She is then gently awakened, the monitors removed, and she is wheeled to recovery a few moments later.

How Will She Feel Afterward?

After a D & C, a woman will experience some cramps and light bleeding for a few days to weeks. If she had a general anesthetic, she may be drowsy and tired for about 24 hours.

If she underwent a D & C for the removal of a nonsurviving pregnancy, the physical symptoms may be overshadowed by her emotions. Women often experience significant grief over the loss of *any* pregnancy, even if they were only pregnant for a few weeks. This can be a complicated reaction, including sadness about the loss and fears about her own ability to carry a normal pregnancy. Guilt, usually unfounded, may be present. These feelings can be made far worse if she suffers from infertility or is nearing the end of her reproductive years. Men often grieve for a pregnancy loss, too.

The D & C is a minor surgical procedure that carries very little risk to our patients. When a D & C is performed, rapid recovery with only minor discomfort is expected. Close cooperation with your partner's doctor and attention to follow-up should lead to excellent results.

What Can I Do to Help?

See the section at the end of the chapter, "Supportive Guy's Recommendations If Your Partner Needs Surgery."

DYSFUNCTIONAL UTERINE BLEEDING

One of the most common problems we see as gynecologists is dysfunctional uterine bleeding (DUB). This is defined as bleeding from the uterus that is *not* caused by uterine abnormalities (e.g., polyps or fibroid tumors) or medical illness (e.g., thyroid disease, blood-clotting problems). Women with DUB are plagued with irregular, unpredictable, and often heavy bleeding. It is especially common at the extremes of reproductive age: in teenagers and women in their 40s. Contributing factors include stress, extreme weight loss or gain, and excessive exercise.

DUB is often the result of the lack of regular ovulation. Recall from Chapter 1 that ovulation is followed by progesterone secretion from the ovary. Progesterone prepares the endometrial lining of the uterus for pregnancy. If pregnancy fails to occur, progesterone levels fall and the lining is shed as a menstrual period. With DUB, ovulation occurs infrequently if at all. Without a menstrual period, the lining continues to build up within the uterus month after month. This fragile tissue then begins to slough off at irregular intervals and sometimes in excessive amounts.

To differentiate DUB from other causes of irregular uterine bleeding, a pelvic exam should be performed. The doctor looks for precancerous tissue or infection in the vagina, cervix, or pelvis that might cause the same symptoms. In addition, lab tests for pregnancy, sex hormone levels, and a thyroid hormone level are often ordered. A biopsy of the uterus, called an endometrial biopsy, may be taken to exclude cancer of the endometrium (the uterine lining). Although not often found in women before the menopause, endometrial cancer may cause the same irregular bleeding as does DUB. In addition, prolonged estrogen stimulation of the uterine lining as seen in DUB can cause this cancer in premenopausal women.

Successful treatment of dysfunctional uterine bleeding can be difficult. The following treatments are often used:

1. **Progestational medications** Medroxyprogesterone acetate (trade name Provera) and other progestational medications can be taken orally for 10 to 12 days each month to help regulate flow.

2. **Estrogen medications** Estrogen medications can be used orally or intravenously to help stop heavy bleeding.

3. **Low-dose birth control pills** Low-dose birth control pills may be used to stop an acute episode of bleeding and/or for long-term prevention of recurrences of irregular bleeding.

4. **Gn RH agonists** New medications known as Gn RH agonists stop estrogen production temporarily through their effect on the pituitary gland (see Chapter 7). When estrogen levels fall, the lining of the uterus stops growing, and bleeding will stop as well.

5. **Surgery** If medical management is unsuccessful, surgical options are available. They include D & C, hysterectomy, and endometrial ablation. Ablation is an outpatient surgical technique in which the lining of the uterus is permanently removed, reducing or stopping any future bleeding (see the section on alternatives to hysterectomy).

SURGERY FOR AN OVARIAN CYST

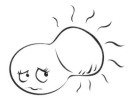 Ovarian cysts are fluid collections within an ovary. They range in size from a few centimeters in diameter to the size of a volleyball! Most ovarian cysts result from normal ovarian function and resolve without treatment. Some continue to grow and require surgical removal. Rarely, ovarian cysts may be premalignant or even cancerous; prompt diagnosis and treatment of these cysts may be lifesaving.

Surgery is necessary for an ovarian cyst when it does not go away on its own, when it is suspected of being cancerous, or when it causes significant pain. Pain may result from rapid growth of the cyst, rupture of the cyst, or from twisting of the enlarged ovary on its stalk (torsion).

 Pain? Picture, if you will, a large fluid-filled sack growing within one of your *testicles*. Now, imagine that cyst tearing open, or the enlarged testicle twisting on its stalk, around and around. Keep this in mind and you'll have no trouble sympathizing when your partner complains of discomfort from a cyst.

Surprisingly, ovarian cysts do not *always* cause pain. It is not uncommon for a woman to have a large ovarian cyst and be unaware of its presence. She may notice only a mild sensation of pressure or a dull ache in the pelvis. It may be uncomfortable to have intercourse or to exercise. Severe pain can occur suddenly from rupture or torsion of the cyst, necessitating a trip to the emergency room.

If an ovarian cyst is present, it will often be detected during a pelvic exam. During this exam, the doctor attempts to feel the uterus and ovaries between his or her hands. An ovarian cyst feels enlarged and soft and is usually tender to the touch.

A cystic ovary can also be identified with a pelvic ultrasound examination. The sonogram helps differentiate an ovarian cyst from other structures within the pelvis. Ovarian cysts can be confused on examination with uterine fibroids, solid ovarian tumors, or swollen loops of intestine.

There are several different types of ovarian cysts. The most common types are:

- **Functional cysts**   Functional cysts are common in women during their reproductive years. Functional cysts result when a follicle keeps growing instead of dissolving after a menstrual cycle (follicles are tiny hormone-producing sacks within the ovary, where eggs mature each month).

- **Polycystic ovarian cysts**   Some women suffer from chronically irregular cycles as a result of disordered hormones and infrequent ovulation. After some time, their ovaries take on a characteristic multicystic appearance. Some of the cysts in women with this condition may grow to several centimeters in diameter.

- **Endometriomas**   As covered in Chapter 7, collections of endometriosis can form cystlike structures on the ovaries. These cysts are lined by endometrial tissue and fill with the blood that tissue produces. Endometriomas are usually painful and can be associated with adhesions (scar tissue) in the pelvis. Endometriomas are seen almost exclusively during a woman's reproductive years. (These are also called "chocolate cysts" because of the dark brown color of the old blood within them.)

- **Dermoid cysts**   These cysts arise from the inner, germ cell layer of the ovary. Dermoid cysts are most common in women ages 20 to 35, and account for 70% of benign ovarian growths in women under 40. Dermoid cysts are benign tumors made of cells from all parts of the body (see below). They do not resolve spontaneously and may grow quite large before they are detected and diagnosed.

 Dermoid cysts arise from the germ cell layer within the ovary. Germ cells are pleuripotent, meaning they can differentiate into any type of cell within the body. Therefore, it is not uncommon for dermoid cysts to contain hair, teeth, skin, and nerves. A dermoid is the likely diagnosis when an ovarian cyst is shown to contain calcified structures (bone, teeth) on X-ray.

- **Cystadenomas** Cystadenomas are tumors that arise from surface cells on the ovary. They will continue to grow until removed and can reach several inches in diameter. They contain either a watery fluid (serous) or thick secretions (mucinous), depending on the type of cell that lines the cyst.

- **Cystic ovarian cancer** Cysts on the ovaries may contain cancer cells. Ovarian cancer occurs with increasing frequency as a woman ages. A woman with a first-degree relative (mother, sister, or daughter) with *certain types* of ovarian or breast cancer may be at higher risk for this disease (ask your doctor). The diagnosis and treatment of ovarian cancer is not covered in this book.

What Are the Alternatives to Surgery?

The only alternative to surgery for a benign-appearing ovarian cyst is to wait for a brief time and see if it goes away on its own. There are few effective treatments; birth control pills may help. Only certain types of ovarian cysts have the potential to resolve spontaneously.

Functional cysts, the most common variety, will usually regress over one to three menstrual cycles. Cysts from poly-cystic ovaries will come and go over time. Endometri-omas, dermoids, cystadenomas, and ovarian cancers will almost always continue to grow until removed. It is important to realize that doctors often don't know for sure which type of cyst is present until *after* surgery.

We know that no one wants an operation they don't need. This fact is balanced with the knowledge that a delay in surgery may result in needless suffering and/or the progression of an early ovarian cancer. Thankfully, the information we obtain about the cyst and our experience leads us to the correct diagnosis before surgery the majority of the time.

The decision to wait or to operate is often complex and must be individualized. Some of the criteria used to make the decision are:

- **Symptoms produced by the cyst**   As mentioned, even a small ovarian cyst may cause severe pain and require surgery immediately. A cyst that causes no symptoms may allow time for observation to see if it goes away on its own.

- **Length of time the cyst has been present**   If the cyst has been present for three or more months/menstrual cycles, it will probably not go away without surgery.

- **Size of the cyst**   A cyst larger than 8 or 10 centimeters (four inches) will probably need to be removed surgically.

- **Bilaterality**   Bilateral cysts (cysts on *both* ovaries) are somewhat more likely to be cancerous and are therefore removed more quickly.

- **Type of cyst**   As mentioned, doctors often don't know for sure what type of cyst is present before surgery. We assemble all the available information, including results from the examination, patient symptoms, and diagnostic test results, and then come up with the most likely diagnosis. If we think she's got a seven-centimeter functional cyst and she's not in pain, we may wait for two to three cycles. If woman has only a four-centimeter cyst but with suspicious test results or a family history putting her at increased risk of ovarian cancer, we might recommend surgery immediately.

What Are the Risks of Surgery?

Once the decision has been made to operate, there are two different approaches: open surgery (laparotomy) and laparoscopic surgery. The approach selected by your gynecologist is determined by several factors, including the type of cyst, the potential need to do other procedures (i.e., hysterectomy) at the same time, and the surgeon's ability to perform laparoscopic surgery.

Laparotomy is the time-honored approach to the treatment of ovarian cysts. The advantages of the open approach are the opportunity to feel as well as look at the pelvic organs, the improved ability to control serious bleeding, and the chance to perform certain procedures that cannot be accomplished through the laparoscope.

Laparoscopy, a newer technique, is performed through small

(half inch) incisions, using a fiber-optic scope and long, narrow instruments. Because of the advances made in instrumentation, this technique has revolutionized surgery in the past 10 years. Many procedures in gynecology, general surgery, and orthopedics—which previously were done only through large open incisions—can be done safely via laparoscopy on an outpatient basis. Laparoscopy's primary advantages when used to treat ovarian cysts are decreased postoperative pain, less scarring in the abdomen after surgery, smaller incisions, and shorter recovery time.

Certain patients, however, may not be good candidates for laparoscopy because of prior surgeries or significant obesity. Other procedures that are planned at the same time may prevent a laparoscopic approach. It may be safer to do a particularly difficult surgery (i.e., remove a large cyst) through a large abdominal incision. If cancer is strongly suspected, open surgery is a better choice for both diagnosing and treating the condition.

The risks of both open surgery and laparoscopy are similar. Each procedure brings with it the risks of bleeding, infection, anesthesia, and damage to surrounding structures. In addition, patients who undergo laparotomy are perhaps more likely to develop adhesions. Adhesions are internal scars that develop wherever tissue was damaged in surgery; they can cause chronic pain or infertility.

A woman who undergoes laparoscopy has a slightly greater risk of injury to the intestines and bladder when compared to open surgery because laparoscopy often requires instruments to be inserted *blindly* through the abdominal wall. These injuries are rare in properly selected patients, and the damage can be completely repaired when recognized. Fewer adhesions *may* result after laparoscopy compared to open surgery because less tissue damage occurs.

What Happens During the Surgery?

If laparotomy is planned, the surgeon makes an incision through the skin of the abdomen. When the cyst is presumed to be benign and the surgery not overly difficult, the incision will usually be low transverse (horizontal). This has also become known as a "bikini" incision because the scar it leaves is nearly invisible to all but the closest of friends. If cancer is suspected or if some other condition that will make the surgery more challenging is present, a vertical skin incision may be used. A vertical incision provides more room to operate once the abdomen is open.

The surgeon uses a scalpel to cut through the muscular and connective tissue layers of the abdominal wall until the abdominal cavity is exposed. As the abdominal cavity is entered, great care is employed to prevent injury to the intestines and bladder. These structures may be adherent (attached) to the abdominal wall from prior surgery or infection. Adhesions on the pelvic organs and/or intestines are removed and the intestines are gently moved out of the way into the upper abdomen.

Once the pelvic organs are adequately displayed, the surgeon inspects the ovaries to confirm the diagnosis of a cyst. The type of the ovarian cyst usually can be determined at this time. The overall health of the other pelvic organs, appendix, liver, gallbladder, intestines, and kidneys is noted. Unless cancer is found, the operation proceeds as planned. If the woman wishes preservation of her ovary, an attempt is made to "shell out" the cyst from the ovary. At times the ovary cannot be separated from the cyst and the ovary and cyst must be removed together. All surgical specimens are sent to the pathologist for microscopic evaluation and final diagnosis. Careful inspection is made to ensure the pelvis is free from bleeding before the abdominal cavity is closed.

The abdomen is closed in layers in the reverse order in which it was opened. Care is taken to remove all instruments and

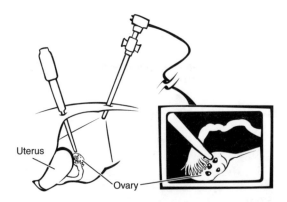

Figure 8.1: *Laparoscopic Video View of the Pelvis*

sponges that were used. The muscular layers are closed thoroughly to ensure a hernia (a gap in the muscular wall surrounding the abdomen) does not develop after surgery. The skin is closed with tiny metal clips or suture and a dressing is applied.

If laparoscopy is to be performed, a narrow instrument is placed through the vagina and into the uterus, which allows the uterus and ovaries to be manipulated during surgery. The surgeon then inserts the laparoscope into the abdominal cavity through a half inch incision just beneath the navel. The abdomen is then filled with CO_2 gas, which lessens the likelihood of injury to the intestines and improves the view of the pelvic organs. A video camera mounted on the laparoscope allows the abdominal and pelvic contents to be seen on a TV monitor in the operating room (see Figure 8.1).

Operating instruments are placed through other small incisions above the pubic bone and/or on each side of the abdomen. A wide variety of excellent instruments are available for grasping, cutting, and cauterizing the pelvic tissues. Needles can be used to drain a cyst before removal. The incisions used and the instruments needed are determined by the surgeon after examination of the pelvis.

Adhesions that obstruct the view of the pelvis or may cause pain are removed. The ovarian cyst is carefully inspected and a diagnosis made. Typically a grasper instrument is used to hold on to the ovary while scissors, graspers, cautery, or laser are used through another incision to remove the cyst. The surgeon follows the entire process on the TV monitors.

Using laparoscopic instruments, the surgeon can remove almost any size or type of ovarian cyst. An ovary can be removed with the cyst if necessary. As in open surgery, all tissues and fluids removed are sent to pathology for final diagnosis.

Extremely large cysts, dense adhesions, excessive bleeding, or findings indicating cancer may cause the laparoscopy to be "converted" to an open surgery. The possibility of conversion to open surgery exists with any laparoscopic procedure.

At the completion of the laparoscopy, the instruments are removed and the CO_2 within the abdomen is allowed to escape. Skin incisions are closed and dressings placed.

Retained CO_2 in the abdomen causes shoulder pain after laparoscopic surgery. This is an example of the phenomenon of *referred pain*—pain that is experienced at a site distant from the actual tissue damage, a result of shared nerve pathways. In this case the pain is actually caused by irritation of the diaphragm. A classic example of referred pain is left arm pain during a heart attack.

Ovarian cysts are very common, but the great majority of them resolve without treatment of any kind. Only a very small percentage of ovarian cysts are cancerous. Careful attention to activity restrictions and follow-up care after surgery are important. A caring and capable physician and your support should bring your partner back to excellent health.

What Can I Do to Help?

See the section at the end of the chapter, "Supportive Guy's Recommendations If Your Partner Needs Surgery."

SURGERY FOR AN ECTOPIC PREGNANCY

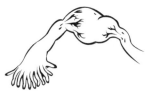

An ectopic pregnancy is a pregnancy that is growing outside of the uterus. Pregnancies cannot survive outside of the uterus, nor can they be placed there if they're growing somewhere else. More than 95% of ectopics occur in the fallopian tube. This is why ectopics are often called tubal pregnancies. The remainder of ectopics are found on an ovary, in the cervix, or in the abdominal cavity.

Fertilization normally occurs outside of the uterus, in the fallopian tube. The sperm "has its way" with the egg at a romantic spot known as the ampulla, at the far end of the fallopian tube.

Under normal circumstances, the happy couple (of sex cells) undergo some intimate cell division for a few days, still in the tube. Then the resulting tiny embryo sashays down the tube into the uterus. The uterine lining (the endometrium) has been prepared during the first two-thirds of the menstrual cycle for just such a visitor. The estrogen and progesterone secreted by the ovary have nourished and stimulated the endometrium, making it lush and thick. Upon arrival, the embryo dives into this most hospitable environment and begins to grow rapidly.

With an ectopic pregnancy, the embryo never implants in the uterus, but attempts to grow somewhere else. Pregnancies growing outside the uterus cannot survive because they cannot get sufficient blood supply for the growing fetus and placenta. Ectopic pregnancies will eventually expire. When the pregnancy dies, internal bleeding often occurs. A pregnancy located anywhere and surviving even for a few weeks has already developed a significant blood supply. As the pregnancy expires, the blood vessels feeding it may tear and bleed, potentially causing major blood loss. In the common case of a tubal ectopic, the fallopian tube may tear and bleed as well; this is referred to as a rupture. Surgery is often needed to prevent or dimish this blood loss and preserve normal pelvic structures. In removing the ectopic pregnancy, a part or all of a fallopian tube or ovary may be lost. Timely diagnosis is important, because it may allow for less invasive surgery or alternative treatments. Ectopic pregnancies, whether located in the tube, cervix, or abdomen, can be life-threatening. It was recently reported that ectopics account for 14% of maternal deaths in the United States.

"As a young resident, I once received an urgent call to evaluate a seriously ill Japanese woman who had just been brought to the emergency room. When I arrived at her bedside, the woman was bent over in severe abdominal pain. Neither she nor her husband spoke any English, and since no one was immediately available to translate, the medical staff could not communicate with her. All they knew was that the woman had been brought by ambulance from a nearby hotel, where she had suddenly collapsed.

She appeared to be in her 30s. She was pale and had a

rapid, shallow pulse. With time for only a brief examination, I noticed that her abdomen was tender and distended (swollen). It was also clear that she was going into shock—her blood pressure was falling and she was losing consciousness.

Blood samples had been drawn the moment she was brought into the emergency room. A blood count, type and crossmatch (for possible transfusion), and a pregnancy test had been sent to the lab. The nurses knew from experience that a woman of her age might well have a complication of pregnancy. As I struggled to make a diagnosis, a "stat" report arrived from the lab: the pregnancy test was positive!

This information brought the whole picture into sharp focus: the woman was suffering from a ruptured ectopic pregnancy.

During OB/GYN training, all residents learn to diagnose this condition. The symptoms include acute lower abdominal pain, dizziness, and vaginal bleeding (may be slight). The physical exam may show falling blood pressure, a rapid pulse, a tender abdomen, and pelvic mass (a swelling or lump where the ectopic is growing). Lab test results will show a positive pregnancy test and a falling blood count. The diagnosis is ruptured ectopic pregnancy with life-threatening internal bleeding, and the treatment plan is immediate surgery.

Through an interpreter who had just arrived, I hurriedly explained to the couple what was happening and what operation was necessary. She was wheeled to an operating room, where, at surgery, more than two liters of blood from a ruptured tubal pregnancy was found in her abdomen. After the involved fallopian tube was removed and a transfusion begun, she stabilized. She recovered nicely and left the hospital in three days.

According to the Centers for Disease Control, the incidence of ectopic pregnancy has been rising, from one in 200 in 1980 to now close to one in 50 pregnancies. In some populations, as many as one in 28 pregnancies is ectopic. The reasons for the rise in rates are an increase in STDs, tubal reconstruction surgery, tubal ligation (sterilization) failures, and complications from previous pelvic infections. All of these factors result in damaged fallopian tubes. An embryo attempting to migrate to the uterus can get trapped in the damaged areas of the tubes.

Are Some Women at Increased Risk for Ectopic Pregnancy?

Risk factors that make a woman more likely to have an ectopic pregnancy are:

- Prior tubal surgery, whether for tubal disease, or to sterilize or reverse prior sterilization surgery;
- Conceiving with an IUD in place (a rare event), because the device prevents normal pregnancies better than it prevents tubal pregnancies;
- Previous episode(s) of pelvic inflammatory disease or endometritis (infection of the uterine lining);
- Use of progestin-only birth control pills;
- Previous ectopic pregnancy.

How is Ectopic Pregnancy Diagnosed?

We attempt to make the diagnosis of an ectopic pregnancy as quickly as we can in order to prevent rupture of the ectopic and bleeding. This can be difficult because symptoms are variable and the diagnostic tests may not be helpful.

The diagnosis of ectopic pregnancy is rarely clear-cut. As physicians, we must be aware of the *possibility* of an ectopic with every early pregnancy, until proven otherwise. Early diagnosis and treatment of ectopic pregnancy has several advantages, and has reduced the mortality of this condition by 90% since 1970.

The textbook symptoms of an ectopic pregnancy are abdominal pain, irregular vaginal bleeding, and a missed period.

Quite often a woman will have few, if any, significant complaints before the abnormal pregnancy ruptures. Many are unaware they are even pregnant when they come in for care.

Blood tests can be helpful in making the diagnosis. A pregnancy test will usually be positive; a blood count may reflect anemia if the woman is bleeding internally.

Pregnancy tests measure a hormone made by the placenta, human chorionic gonadotrophin (Beta-HCG). With a normal early pregnancy, the level of Beta-HCG will double approximately every two days. With an ectopic pregnancy, the levels are usually lower than expected and rise more slowly, if at all.

If a pregnant woman is suspected of having an ectopic pregnancy, she may be asked to have her blood tested for Beta-HCG level for a few days to see if it is rising normally. Although this is often helpful in making a diagnosis of ectopic pregnancy, matters are complicated by the fact that some ectopics initially show normal doubling of Beta-HCG levels, and some normal pregnancies do not.

An ultrasound examination of the pelvis may exclude the diagnosis of ectopic pregnancy by demonstrating that the pregnancy is in the uterus. The pregnancy should be visible by five to six weeks after the start of the last menstrual period, or three to four weeks after conception. On rare occasions, a sonogram will actually show a pregnancy that is developing *outside* of the uterus.

About once in every 10,000 pregnancies, a woman will have an intrauterine pregnancy and an ectopic pregnancy simultaneously. This happens more often in women taking fertility medications. It can be particularly dangerous, since the ectopic is rarely suspected once the normal pregnancy is identified.

A recent advance in ultrasound is the vaginal probe. It can be placed up against the cervix via the vagina, creating a much more detailed ultrasound image than that supplied from an external probe (see figure 8.2). This direct view enables the gynecologist to identify a pregnancy within the uterus at less than six weeks of pregnancy. It's a very important tool in the early diagnosis of ectopic pregnancy.

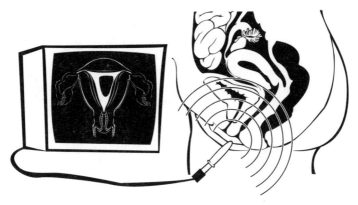

Figure 8.2: Vaginal Probe

The only way to be certain a woman has an ectopic pregnancy (unless it's seen on ultrasound) is to find it during surgery. Since this involves risk, we try to make the diagnosis with other, less invasive methods, if possible.

A D & C may be performed before laparoscopy to help exclude the diagnosis of ectopic pregnancy. If we know the pregnancy is abnormal, a D & C can tell us if pregnancy tissue is inside the uterus; if it is found there, the laparoscopy can then be avoided.

Do Ectopic Pregnancies Cause Long-Term Problems?

In addition to the immediate problems caused by an ectopic pregnancy, important long-term concerns also arise. Women who have suffered an ectopic may become infertile as a result of tubal damage that occurred. Women with the best chance for future fertility after an ectopic have no other fertility problems and a normal-appearing opposite fallopian tube at surgery. A second ectopic pregnancy occurs approximately 15% of the time when pregnancy is re-attempted.

In a recent study, 110 patients were followed after they had ectopic pregnancies. All were interested in becoming pregnant again. Sixty-five percent had subsequent normal pregnancies, 22% had repeat ectopics, and 15% remained infertile. Other studies have shown that between 20 and 60% of women who have had two ectopics have normal pregnancies afterward.

J. I. Mackinen et al., *International Journal of Fertility* 34(1): 46–51 (1989).

What Are the Alternatives to Surgery?

If the diagnosis of ectopic pregnancy is made early and the patient is without significant bleeding or pain, three different approaches to treatment may be available: surgery, expectant management, and medical therapy.

The first approach to the treatment of an ectopic is to surgically remove it. If surgery is to be performed, there are additional choices: removing only the ectopic and leaving the tube behind, removing the ectopic and the involved segment of tube, or removing the entire fallopian tube that contains the ectopic. The next section details these choices.

A nonsurgical treatment option is close observation, called expectant management. This option is not open to many women. It is reserved for the unusual case of a woman with a small ectopic (size can sometimes be determined through ultrasound measurement), few or no symptoms, a stable blood count, and falling levels of the pregnancy hormone (Beta-HCG). In these cases, a woman may need nothing more than restriction of activity and close follow-up. Exercise and sex must avoided, as they can lead to rupture. Over a few days to weeks, successful expectant management allows an ectopic pregnancy to expire and be resorbed by the body. This result can be confirmed through levels of Beta-HCG that fall to zero and the disappearance of the patient's symptoms.

A risk during expectant management is the sudden rupture of the ectopic pregnancy. This can happen with any size of ectopic, causing sudden internal bleeding. As mentioned, this can be dangerous, even life-threatening.

Sixty-seven women with stable ectopic pregnancies were followed expectantly in a recent report. Forty-nine of the women (73%) had spontaneous resolution of their pregnancies, 15 needed surgery for signs of rupture, and 3 had medical treatment. The best success with expectant management was achieved by women with a low level of Beta-HCG, a small ectopic, and minimal bleeding and pain.

D. Trio et al., "Prognostic factors for successful expectant management of ectopic pregnancy," *Fertility and Sterility* 63: 469–472 (1995).

Another nonsurgical alternative for treating ectopic pregnancies is medical therapy. The use of medications to treat ectopics has advanced greatly in the past decade. Various medicines have been studied, including potassium chloride and prostaglandin (a hormone that causes tubal contractions) injected directly into the fallopian tube, RU-486, and the anticancer drug methotrexate.

The best results have been achieved with methotrexate. Used also to treat psoriasis, arthritis, and some types of cancer, this drug attacks the rapidly dividing cells found in an ectopic pregnancy. Candidates in our hospital for methotrexate treatment are patients with no internal bleeding and a small ectopic (no larger than three and a half centimeters) and without a visible heartbeat on ultrasound. Lab tests show normal liver and kidney function and a normal blood count. Prior tubal sterilization surgery precludes the use of methotrexate. Properly selected patients are successfully treated with this medication more than 90% of the time.

Methotrexate is given as a single intramuscular injection. Rare side effects include mouth sores, flu-like symptoms, and liver inflammation. Once the medication has been given, the woman can be sent home. She is instructed to return for follow-up testing of Beta-HCG levels until they fall to zero, which takes two to six weeks. She is also told to avoid strenuous exercise or intercourse and to report any unusual symptoms. On occasion, repeat doses of methotrexate may be needed.

Crucial to the safety and success of methotrexate treatment are the following:

- **Proper patient selection**   Women with large ectopics or high levels of Beta-HCG have a greater chance of not responding to the medical treatment and needing surgery.

- **Avoidance of certain medications**   Prenatal vitamins, aspirin, folic acid, phenytoin, sulfa-containing drugs, and alcohol cannot be taken until the pregnancy test result is negative. They interfere with the action of methotrexate.

- **Attention to activity restrictions**   Until the pregnancy has completely resolved, strenuous exercise and intercourse must be avoided. Rupture and internal bleeding could occur at any time.

- **Close follow-up blood testing and immediate reporting of heavy bleeding, dizziness, or severe pain**

As mentioned, in properly selected women with ectopics the chances of successful treatment with methotrexate are excellent. Side effects are mild and rarely seen, and no increase in birth defects with subsequent pregnancies has been noted. The chances of having another ectopic appear to be no higher after this form of treatment than for those women who have surgery.

Ectopic pregnancy has almost always required surgery in the past. The addition of methotrexate, a highly effective, nonsurgical alternative, has been welcomed by both patients and doctors. For the right patients, the pain and risks of surgery can be avoided, as can the costs of hospitalization.

What Are the Risks of Surgery?

As mentioned earlier in the chapter, all operations carry the same basic risks: infection, bleeding, damage to internal structures, and complications from anesthesia.

If surgery is necessary for an ectopic pregnancy, there are two approaches: open surgery (laparotomy) and laparoscopy, through two to four tiny incisions. As in the case of an ovarian cyst, the type of surgical approach is based on many factors. With an ectopic pregnancy, some of these factors are:

- **Size of the ectopic**   Larger ectopics tend to bleed more during surgery and may be more safely managed through an open abdominal incision.

- **Presence of internal bleeding**   Hemorrhage may obscure the view through the laparoscope. Life-threatening bleeding (leading to shock) with an ectopic requires the quickest approach: an open abdominal incision.

- **Patient's suitability for laparoscopy** Women who are either excessively overweight or who have had multiple prior surgeries and scarring may not be candidates for the laparoscopic approach. Injuries to internal organs or other operative complications are more likely in these patients.

- **Surgeon's level of expertise with laparoscopy and availability of equipment**

One important risk of a surgical approach to the treatment of an ectopic is that some of the pregnancy may be left behind in the fallopian tube. This complication is called a "persistent ectopic." Persistent ectopics are found 5 to 10% of the time after conservative surgery, when the tube containing the ectopic is not entirely removed. This occurs most commonly after laparoscopy. Since persistent ectopics have the capacity to cause significant internal bleeding and tubal damage, they are treated aggressively with either surgery or methotrexate. Recent studies have investigated whether giving methotrexate immediately after conservative tubal surgery can lower rates of persistent ectopics; preliminary results are encouraging.*

If a woman is treated surgically for an ectopic without removing the entire fallopian tube, she must have follow-up to ensure that a persistent ectopic isn't developing. Besides the usual postoperative precautions, she will need to have regular blood tests for Beta-HCG levels to prove the pregnancy has been entirely removed. Even if she's feeling better, she may have a persistent ectopic.

What Happens During the Surgery?

If we know the pregnancy isn't normal but we're not sure where it is, we often start with a D & C. With this procedure, we can find out if the pregnancy is in the uterus. The tissue from the uterus is sent to the pathologist. If pregnancy tissue is found, this usually excludes the diagnosis of ectopic pregnancy and the operation is terminated.

---

*J. W. Graczykowski and D. R. Mishell, "Methotrexate prophylaxis for persistent ectopic pregnancy after conservative treatment by salpingostomy," *Obstetrics and Gynecology* 89: 118 (1997).

Often it is necessary to perform either open surgery or laparoscopy to detect an ectopic pregnancy (the basic approach to these techniques has been described previously in this chapter). If an ectopic pregnancy is identified, the surgery proceeds in one of the following ways:

1. **Salpingostomy** Open the fallopian tube, remove the ectopic, close the tube (or let it close on its own).

2. **Partial salpingectomy** Remove the part of the tube that has the ectopic. The two ends of the tube can sometimes be reconnected later.

3. **Salpingectomy** Remove the entire tube that contains the ectopic.

The surgeon chooses which type of surgery to perform based on the condition of the tubes and the woman's wishes for future fertility. All of these surgical procedures can be done through the laparoscope or via an abdominal incision in most cases.

The problem of ectopic pregnancy is increasingly common. Most women with ectopics do not have any of the risk factors outlined earlier. Thankfully, improved methods of diagnosis have led to a sharp decrease in emergency surgery and deaths. Early diagnosis also allows for more treatment options and improved future fertility. If you and your mate are confronted by an ectopic pregnancy, competent medical care and your cooperation should lead to a healthy outcome.

What Can I Do to Help?

See the section at the end of the chapter, "Supportive Guy's Recommendations If Your Partner Needs Surgery."

HYSTERECTOMY

"It will be a year since my hysterectomy. What a great operation! I'm indebted to you forever. My menstrual suffering is over . . . Thank you, thank you, thank you."

— N. S., San Diego, CA

"We wouldn't be having sex if it wasn't for my hysterectomy."

— P. M., Coronado, CA

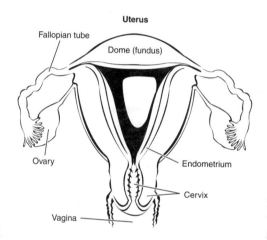

Hysterectomy is the surgical removal of the uterus. By reading *Your Guy's Guide to Gynecology*, you've already learned much about this amazing organ: the uterus is the site where a fetus grows during pregnancy; composed primarily of muscle tissue, its contractions during labor expel the newborn baby; when no pregnancy exists, the inner lining of the uterus (the endometrium) is shed each month as a menstrual period; the vaginal entrance to the uterus is the cervix, which dilates to allow the birth of a baby. A Pap smear is a test of the cervix for cancer.

To really understand hysterectomy, you also need to know that we are talking about removing a woman's *womb*. This organ is often of great emotional and spiritual significance. Some women believe they will suffer significant changes in their sexuality or lose their desirability and femininity if they have a hysterectomy. Regardless, to remove the uterus for any reason will be a major event in any woman's life.

There are several different types of hysterectomy. A partial or subtotal hysterectomy removes the body of the uterus but leaves the cervix. (Some people may incorrectly use the term *partial hysterectomy* to mean removal of the uterus without removal of the ovaries.) A complete or total hysterectomy means removal of the entire uterus and cervix. A radical hysterectomy, done to treat cancer, requires taking out the uterus, cervix, and surrounding supportive ligaments and tissues; often, the ovaries and tubes are removed as well.

Hysterectomies also vary by the route through which the organ is removed. The uterus can be removed through an abdominal or vaginal incision. These types of hysterectomy, as well as other procedures commonly done at the same time, will be covered later in this section.

 How common is hysterectomy? It has been reported to be the second most common surgery in America. Recently, a study found that one of three women in the United States had had a hysterectomy by the age of 60. In the past few years, many new medical and surgical treatments have been taking the place of hysterectomy.

R. Pokras et al., "Hysterectomies in the U.S., 1965–1984," National Center for Health Statistics, Vital Health Statistics Series 13, No. 92, Department of Health and Human Services, Pub. No. (PHS) 87–1753 (1987).

Hysterectomies are done for a variety of reasons. The most common (in decreasing order) are:

- **Uterine fibroids**   A hysterectomy may be performed to remove fibroids that are causing heavy bleeding, pain, and/or pressure.

- **Endometriosis**   A hysterectomy may be performed to treat endometriosis causing chronic pain and/or irregular bleeding.

- **Uterine prolapse**   If the supportive ligaments of the uterus have weakened, the uterus may fall into the vagina or, in some cases, almost completely out of the vagina. In these cases, a hysterectomy may be needed.

- **Cancer**   Cancer of the uterus, cervix, or ovaries may require a hysterectomy.

- **Endometrial hyperplasia**   Precancerous changes of the uterine lining may require a hysterectomy.

- **Menstrual/menopausal symptoms**   Irregular and/or prolonged bleeding not responsive to medications or minor surgery may be treated using hysterectomy.

- **Cervical dysplasia**   Severe precancerous changes of the cervix may be treated with a hysterectomy.

- **Pelvic pain** Pelvic pain believed to be related to the uterus may require a hysterectomy.

What Are the Alternatives to Hysterectomy?

Hysterectomy is a major operation and carries significant risks. It is also a major emotional event for a woman and her family. Because of advances in medical and minor surgical treatments of many disorders that affect the uterus, hysterectomy can often be delayed or avoided altogether. In many cases, however, a hysterectomy may bring a great improvement in quality of life or may even be lifesaving.

Alternative Treatments for Uterine Fibroids

Uterine fibroids are the most common reason for hysterectomy. As discussed in Chapter 7, fibroids are benign (noncancerous) muscular tumors of the uterus. They can range in size from a few millimeters to the size of a large melon. Fibroids are often multiple and can be found within the wall of the uterus, in the endometrial cavity, or attached to the outside of the uterus on a stalk (see Figure 8.3). They may or may not produce symptoms, depending on their size and location.

Symptoms of uterine fibroids may include heavy menstrual flow, irregular bleeding, cramps, pelvic pain or pressure, discomfort with intercourse, low back pain, frequent urination, or difficulty with bowel movements.

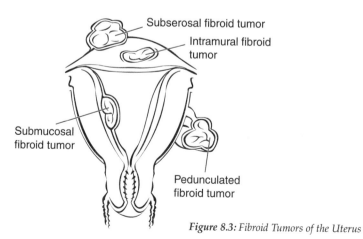

Subserosal fibroid tumor

Intramural fibroid tumor

Submucosal fibroid tumor

Pedunculated fibroid tumor

Figure 8.3: Fibroid Tumors of the Uterus

Until recently, a hysterectomy was recommended for a woman if her fibroids enlarged the uterus enough to fill the pelvis (about the size of a twelve-week pregnancy) even if her fibroids didn't cause symptoms. It was believed that a uterus of this size required surgery because doctors could no longer reliably detect ovarian growth that might mean cancer. In addition, since fibroids typically grow over time, further delay would result in a larger uterus and a more difficult and risky operation.

Ultrasound examination of the pelvis has now made it possible to detect ovarian changes, in most cases, regardless of the size of the uterus. Ultrasound also provides more information about the ovaries than can be gained from a pelvic exam. Certain features of ovarian growth are more suggestive of cancer than others and cannot be determined as reliably on pelvic exam as they can with ultrasound.

The increasing use of ultrasound should reduce the number of hysterectomies being performed for fibroids in women without symptoms.

In women with fibroids who have heavy and/or irregular periods, there may be other treatment approaches aside from hysterectomy. Abnormal bleeding can sometimes be managed successfully with oral progesterone derivatives, progesterone injections (trade name Depo-Provera), or birth control pills. However, for some women these approaches are inadequate or provide only temporary relief of their symptoms. Fibroids usually continue to grow over time, as does their capacity to cause problems.

As described in Chapter 7, a woman suffering from fibroids may be offered medical treatment with Gn RH agonists, a new class of medications that rapidly lower estrogen levels. Since fibroids are estrogen-dependent, this causes them to shrink significantly, in three to six months. Many of the symptoms caused by the fibroids will diminish or disappear as they decrease in size. Unfortunately, there are often side effects from the low estrogen levels: hot flashes, insomnia, and vaginal dryness. Another problem with Gn RH medications is that they cause thinning of the bones (osteoporosis) if used for more than six months. Stopping the medication results in re-growth of the fibroids, so Gn RH agonists do not represent a cure. Current research is investigating whether a small amount of estrogen and/or progesterone replacement can make the side effects of Gn RH agonists more tolerable and protect the bones while allowing prolonged treatment.

New minor surgery approaches can often help women with fibroids when medicines don't. When compared to hysterectomy, these treatments offer retention of the uterus, a shorter hospital stay, lower cost, and a more rapid return to full activity.

Fibroids within the cavity of the uterus can often be removed with a technique called hysteroscopy. Hysteroscopic removal of fibroids is an outpatient procedure. A narrow fiber-optic scope is passed through the cervix of an anesthetized woman so the gynecologist can see the inside of the uterine cavity. Fibroids or polyps (overgrown glands) can be removed with specialized instruments while the doctor watches through the scope. Pretreatment for two to three months with Gn RH agonists to shrink large fibroids may make their removal easier.

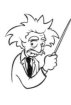

In a study of the effectiveness of the removal of fibroids with hysteroscopy in New York between 1988 and 1994, 94% of 120 women had normal menstrual flow six months after the procedure. Eighty-four percent of the women were still satisfied six years after the surgery. Less than five percent had major operative complications, and fewer than 10% needed additional surgery within six months.

D. R. Phillips et al., "Transcervical electro-resection of submucous myomas for chronic menorrhagia," *Journal of the American Association of Gynecological Laparoscopy*, 2(2): 147–53 (1995).

Another use of hysteroscopy in the treatment of abnormal bleeding is endometrial ablation. In this technique, an electro-surgical or laser instrument attached to the hysteroscope removes or destroys the endometrial lining. Once the endometrial lining is gone, there will be little or no menstrual flow. Before surgery, the patient is often given Gn RH agonists to thin the endometrium and improve the surgical result. Endometrial ablation, accompanied by hysteroscopic removal of fibroids, will significantly decrease or even eliminate monthly periods.

In the largest study to date, 600 laser ablations were performed in the United Kingdom for heavy menstrual bleeding. The women were given medications preoperatively to thin their endometrium. Fifteen months later, 83% judged their surgery a success. There were no major operative complications.

R. Garry et al., "Six hundred endometrial laser ablations," *Obstetrics and Gynecology* 85: 24–29 (1995).

As with all treatment options, ablation has its shortcomings. Although *extremely* unlikely, women who become pregnant after ablation seem to have a higher risk of an ectopic pregnancy. In addition, a very small risk of endometrial cancer remains if any lining tissue is left inside the uterus after the surgery, and early detection may be hindered because evaluation of the uterine cavity is more difficult after ablation.

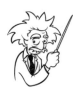

Of interest is another recent study that followed women with ablation and standard total hysterectomy for two years. The women who had ablation expressed more dissatisfaction (21% versus 4%) even though they had much less invasive surgery. They complained of more pain, more emotional problems, and overall a poorer quality of life than those who had undergone hysterectomy.

M. J. Sculphers et al., "Randomized trial comparing hysterectomy and transcervical endometrial ablation; Effect on health related quality of life and costs 2 years post op," *British Journal of Obstetrics and Gynecology* 103(2): 142–9 (1996).

Complications of hysteroscopy include those mentioned previously: bleeding, infection, anesthesia, and damage to surrounding organs. In addition, fluid overload may occur, causing sudden respiratory or cardiac problems. (This occurs because fluid is slowly pumped into the uterus during the surgery to help the surgeon see.) Hysteroscopy is generally a very safe procedure when patients are appropriately chosen and cared for during and after surgery.

Currently, new instruments and techniques are being evaluated that may make ablation quicker and easier to perform. These new approaches may be safer as well.

A new approach to ablation that is quicker and potentially

safer is called "ThermaChoice." With this technique, the endometrium is destroyed by heating it with a balloon filled with sterile fluid. Preliminary results show effectiveness similar to other ablation methods, and the process takes just eight minutes once the balloon is inserted.

Myomectomy is another alternative to hysterectomy in women with fibroids. Myomectomy is the surgical removal of fibroids that are within the wall of the uterus or on its surface. It is most often done through an abdominal incision (laparotomy), but in certain cases it may be done through the laparoscope.

The appeal of myomectomy is that it removes the abnormal tissue (the fibroids) while retaining the uterus. Women who wish to have children or simply to keep their uterus may be candidates for this procedure.

Myomectomy may be more difficult and risky than a hysterectomy. Although less tissue is removed in a myomectomy than in a hysterectomy, data show that myomectomy carries a higher risk of significant bleeding and infection. Fibroids are muscular tumors with a rich blood supply. The greater the number and the larger the size of the fibroids, the more difficult the operation. Uncontrolled bleeding during myomectomy may require an emergency hysterectomy. Women are often treated with Gn RH agonists for two to three months before surgery to shrink the fibroids and decrease bleeding at surgery. Donating one to two units of blood before myomectomy, just in case, is not a bad idea.

An additional risk of myomectomy is the formation of pelvic adhesions (scar tissue) after the operation. Adhesions can sometimes cause pelvic pain or infertility. In addition, damage to the bowels, bladder, fallopian tubes, and ureters (which drain the kidneys) may occur. Most important, fibroids often recur after myomectomy and may require additional surgery.

It is estimated that 20 to 50% of women will have regrowth of fibroids after myomectomy, often requiring hysterectomy.

A woman with fibroids who wishes to keep her uterus may be a candidate for myomectomy. Myomectomy may be performed when the following are present:

- heavy menstrual bleeding not responsive to medical therapy;
- rapid growth of fibroid(s);
- recurrent pregnancy loss caused by a distorted uterine cavity (from fibroids);
- obstruction of nearby organs, such as the fallopian tubes, the bladder, the intestines, or the ureters;
- infertility (in the absence of other factors).

Alternative Treatments for Other Problems

Alternative treatments may exist for some of the other indications for hysterectomy as well. Briefly, the indications and their alternatives are as follows:

- **Endometriosis**   Medical treatment with Gn RH agonists, progestins, anti-estrogens, and oral contraceptives may provide relief. Laparoscopy or open surgery with electro-surgical or laser treatment of endometriosis is often effective in treating the pain caused by this disease.

- **Uterine prolapse**   Women suffering from significant "pelvic relaxation" may have multiple symptoms: feeling a bulge in the vagina from the uterus falling down, urinary incontinence, and difficulty with bowel movements. If her problems are minor or if she doesn't want surgery, she may be treated with a pessary. These plastic or rubber devices are made to fit in the vagina comfortably and help support the uterus. Kegel's exercises may strengthen the pelvic floor muscles when used consistently.

  Note: not all urinary incontinence is caused by relaxation of the pelvic floor; a thorough evaluation is required of any incontinence before surgery is planned.

- **Cancer of the cervix, uterus, or ovaries**   These diseases are life-threatening and hysterectomy is often the best treatment. However, other options may be available depending on the specific type of cancer and how much it has spread. A detailed description of these cancers and their treatment is beyond the scope of this book. A gynecologic oncologist is trained to address these concerns.

- **Endometrial hyperplasia**   The consequences of inadequate treatment of this precancer may be dire, but individual cases can sometimes be safely treated with hormonal medications (progestins). Close follow-up is necessary to ensure the disease has not recurred or progressed to cancer.

*   **Menstrual/menopausal symptoms** This refers primarily to bleeding difficulties. The use of progesterone derivatives such as Depo-Provera may provide relief. Birth control pills are often recommended and have additional health benefits for many women in their 40s. In addition, hysteroscopy with endometrial ablation may be an effective treatment.

*   **Cervical dysplasia** This disease can often be treated with minor surgery. (See the section in Chapter 7 for more details.)

*   **Pelvic pain** Before resorting to hysterectomy, most women with pelvic pain undergo treatment with various medications. Laparoscopy or less extensive surgery may also relieve their pain. Some women also respond very well to biofeedback and/or counseling.

Alternative approaches to hysterectomy often exist. Don't be afraid to ask your partner's doctor about them, but remember: hysterectomy can bring a big improvement in the quality of her life and may even be lifesaving. The choice is an individual one and should be made only after getting familiar with the problem(s) as well as any other treatment options.

What Are the Risks of Hysterectomy?

Hysterectomy is a major operation. The previously noted risks of surgery certainly apply, including bleeding, infection, and anesthesia. Injury to the intestines and/or bladder also may occur.

An additional risk that applies to hysterectomy (and all major surgeries) is the formation of blood clots in the legs during or after the surgery. This risk increases with the length of time the operation takes, with the amount of tissue damaged during surgery, and if cancer is found.

Blood clots can travel to the lungs and obstruct blood flow (see "the professor" below). Being in one position for a long period of time, along with the tissue damage that occurs with surgery, increase the risk of this life-threatening complication. The gynecologist may prescribe medication and/or special stockings during and after surgery to prevent blood clots.

Blood clots can form *any time* you stay in one position for too long, even without surgery. The fancy medical name for them is deep venous thromboses (DVTs). When the clots move to the lungs, they obstruct the circulation and can be lethal. These are called pulmonary emboli.

A gynecologic surgeon will bring a woman through her hysterectomy with flying colors in the vast majority of cases. However, complications are not always preventable, even when the patient is in the best of hands. You may want to ask the doctor how many hysterectomies he or she has done, as well as how often transfusions were necessary or complications occurred during previous surgeries. In the vast majority of cases, these answers will be reassuring. Seeking a second opinion is a good idea if it makes you more comfortable before surgery. This is even required by some insurance companies.

What Happens During the Surgery?

Operative Approaches

There are two basic operative approaches to hysterectomy: abdominal and vaginal. About three-fourths of all hysterectomies currently are done abdominally (the uterus is removed through an abdominal incision). A third type of hysterectomy is also done. It is called LAVH, which stands for laparoscopically assisted vaginal hysterectomy. This new operation is a hybrid of the vaginal hysterectomy and laparoscopic surgery.

The LAVH allows a woman to have a primarily vaginal operation (with quicker healing) instead of an abdominal one. One reason women often had a hysterectomy via the abdominal approach was because this was the safest way to remove pelvic adhesions (from old infections or prior surgery). Newer laparoscopic techniques used during an LAVH make it possible to cut these adhesions without opening the abdomen, in most cases.

Another important reason for the abdominal approach to hysterectomy was to ensure safe removal of the ovaries and/or fallopian tubes. This can now usually be accomplished with the advanced laparoscopic instruments used during an LAVH.

In the current climate of cost savings, the vaginal hysterectomy and LAVH have an edge over abdominal surgery. From the perspective of the insurance companies, vaginal surgery allows a patient to be discharged earlier, which saves money. In addition, vaginal surgery leads to quicker recovery at home and an earlier return to her job (which may or *may not* make her happy). On average, she can engage in most activities three to four weeks after a vaginal hysterectomy or LAVH, compared to six weeks with abdominal surgery.

An abdominal hysterectomy requires a large abdominal incision, either low transverse or low vertical. The scar that remains is initially quite painful and ultimately very permanent. LAVH leaves much smaller abdominal scars, and vaginal surgery uses no abdominal incisions.

Not all hysterectomies can be done safely by the vaginal or LAVH route. Endometriosis, prior surgery, or infection may have caused pelvic adhesions so severe that an open incision is necessary to complete the operation. Women with a very narrow pelvis and/or a well-supported uterus may not be good candidates, either, because it would be too technically difficult. Large fibroid tumors may prevent vaginal removal of the uterus.

Recently, Gn RH agonists have been used to "convert" some women from needing an abdominal hysterectomy to having a LAVH or a vaginal hysterectomy. Pretreatment with these medications for three to six months before surgery often shrinks the fibroids enough to allow vaginal surgery. In addition, this delay often allows women to raise their blood counts by taking iron supplements, which lowers their risk of needing a transfusion.

In a recent study, a group of researchers used a Gn RH agonist to shrink fibroids in women with very large uteri. Overall, about 50% of the women were able to have vaginal surgery after the pretreatment. Their length of stay in the hospital and total recovery times were significantly shorter than the women who had abdominal hysterectomies.

T. G. Stovall et al., *American Journal of Obstetrics and Gynecology* 70: 1744–1751 (1999).

The decision of whether to remove the ovaries and fallopian tubes must always be made when a hysterectomy is planned. This is a highly individual decision that should be discussed with your partner's doctor. If the ovaries and tubes are removed before the menopause, the woman will experience the effects of a rapid fall in her estrogen levels. The most common symptoms of this "surgical menopause" are hot flashes, vaginal dryness, and insomnia. As we detailed in Chapter 6, estrogen in small doses will often relieve these symptoms.

On the other hand, if her ovaries are removed at the time of her hysterectomy, she will never again have to face surgery for problems with her ovaries, including ovarian cancer. Some women are at high risk for ovarian cancer.

In general, we don't recommend removal of the ovaries and tubes unless:

- The ovaries and/or tubes are involved with the disease process, as with endometriosis (much higher rates of recurrent pain and re-operation are found if the ovaries are retained) or cancer.

- The woman is over 45 years old: the ovaries are not expected to produce estrogen for more than a few more years but the chance of developing cancer or other diseases of the ovaries remains.

- There is a family history of cancer that increases her risk of ovarian cancer.

- The woman requests removal of her ovaries and tubes at the time of her hysterectomy.

Aside from removal of the ovaries and tubes, other procedures may be done at the time of hysterectomy. Correction of pelvic support problems (urinary incontinence surgery, repair of bladder, intestine, or rectal support), removal of scar tissue, and even appendectomy (removal of the appendix) may be as important as the hysterectomy itself.

Recently, there has been a resurgence in interest in preserving the cervix when a hysterectomy is planned. The primary motive is a belief that sexual function is better preserved if the cervix is left behind. Until definitive research is done, "subtotal hysterectomy" will not be standard practice, but is an acceptable option for women without abnormal pap smears or other diseases affecting the cervix. From a practical standpoint, this request would also prevent her doctor from doing a vaginal hysterectomy, since that approach mandates removal of the cervix. Either an abdominal or laparoscopic approach would be necessary.

The decision to perform a hysterectomy is not the only one to be made. The surgical approach (abdominal, vaginal, or LAVH), as well as the need for other procedures, will need to be discussed with your partner's gynecologist. Specific surgical procedures for each approach are discussed below.

Sometimes a particular type of hysterectomy is clearly better for a woman despite her desire for another. Some women request surgery but we discourage them because alternate treatments would be safer and/or just as effective. Occasionally women resist a hysterectomy because of fears of the effects it will have later on.

It is important to set aside some time with your doctor to talk through all of these points until the treatment plan is understandable and agreeable to both of you. If agreement is difficult to come by, a second opinion may be of some help. These discussions should take place well before the day of surgery.

Abdominal Hysterectomy

Removal of the uterus through the abdomen is accomplished in a careful and systematic fashion. Hysterectomy technique may vary slightly depending on where a physician trained and his or her level of experience. The exact approach is also affected by the condition of the pelvic organs and the other procedures planned. For a straightforward abdominal hysterectomy, these general statements can be made:

• After induction of anesthesia and sterile preparation of the abdominal skin, the abdomen is opened layer by layer through a low transverse or vertical incision.

• Once the abdominal cavity is opened, the gynecologic surgeon and his or her assistant explore it to confirm the diagnosis (e.g., fibroids, endometriosis) and inspect the other organs (stomach, liver, kidneys, etc.). Care is taken throughout the operation to avoid damaging surrounding structures, specifically the intestines, ureters, bladder, and blood vessels.

• The intestines are gently moved into the upper abdomen to optimize the exposure of the pelvis. Any scar tissue (adhesions) that affects the pelvic organs or intestines is removed.

• The surgeons methodically remove the attachments and blood supply to the uterus. The supportive ligaments are clamped and cut from the top of the uterus down toward the cervix and tied with suture to secure them.

• The bladder is released from its position on the lower portion of the uterus and pushed gently down and out of the way.

• The uterus is detached by cutting between the cervix and the top of the vagina. It is sent to the pathologist for inspection and final diagnosis. The vaginal opening is sewn closed in a way that its diameter and length are not compromised.

• The pelvis is carefully inspected for bleeding; additional sutures and/or cautery are used as needed.

• The abdomen is carefully closed in layers, to ensure good healing. The skin is closed with suture or clips, and a dressing is applied.

Vaginal Hysterectomy

• After induction of anesthesia and sterile preparation of the vagina, an incision is made around the cervix where it meets the vagina.

• A small opening is carefully made into the abdominal cavity beneath the uterus.

• The supportive ligaments of the uterus are clamped, cut, and tied with suture from the bottom up (the reverse of abdominal hysterectomy).

• After some of the ligaments at the base of the uterus have been freed, an opening into the abdominal cavity is made above the uterus and beneath the bladder.

• Clamps are placed completely around the tissue that supports the uterus. The tissue in the clamps is cut and tied. Successive "bites" of tissue are taken until the uterus is free. Once the uterus is detached, it can be gently pulled down and out through the vagina. It is sent to the pathologist for examination.

• The sutured tissue is inspected for bleeding, and then the openings in the abdominal cavity and vagina are sewn closed. Often a packing (gauze) is placed into the vagina and left there until the following morning to help minimize bleeding.

Laparoscopically Assisted Vaginal Hysterectomy

The laparoscopically assisted vaginal hysterectomy is a two-stage operation. The surgery is begun through the laparoscope, with the surgeon looking into the abdominal cavity. It is completed through the vagina. Again, technique varies somewhat from surgeon to surgeon; some do more and some less through the laparoscope before moving to the vaginal part. What follows is our standard approach:

• After induction of anesthesia and sterile preparation of the abdomen and vagina, the laparoscope is inserted beneath the umbilicus (belly button), displaying the pelvic and abdominal contents. A second instrument is placed to one side of the laparoscope through another small incision.

• The intestines are moved into the upper abdomen, and the pelvis is inspected to see if the woman can safely have an

LAVH. Any scar tissue (adhesions) involving the pelvis or intestines is cut.

• An instrument using either permanent staples or electric current is inserted through another small incision and is used to divide the tissue between the uterus and the ovaries and tubes. These highly advanced instruments also prevent bleeding in the divided tissue. The same instrument is used to divide the supportive ligaments of the uterus down toward the cervix.

• Using a tiny scissors with electrical current, a cut is made between the bladder and the lower part of the uterus. The incision is extended across the junction of the bladder and uterus. The bladder can then be pushed gently away from the uterus.

• The remainder of the surgery is completed vaginally, where an incision is made between the cervix and the vagina. As in vaginal hysterectomy, an entrance is made below the uterus into the abdominal cavity.

• The lower ligaments of the uterus are then clamped, cut, and tied from below. An entrance into the abdominal cavity above the cervix is made. The rest of the tissue holding the uterus is clamped and cut, and it is removed through the vaginal opening. The uterus is sent to the pathologist for final diagnosis.

• The tissues are inspected for bleeding, and then the openings in the pelvis and vagina are sewn closed.

• Before completing the procedure, the laparoscope is once again used to inspect the pelvis for bleeding. All instruments are removed, the abdominal incisions are closed, and dressings are applied.

What Can I Do to Help?

A recent study concluded that the availability of a supportive confidant provided protection from depression in post-hysterectomy patients.* So, supportive mates have now been scientifically proven to help in the recovery process after hysterectomy.

However, according to a popular gynecology textbook, "as unaware as women may be about the functioning of their

---

*C. Webb, "Professional and lay support for hysterectomy patients," *Journal of Advanced Nursing* 11: 167 (1986).

bodies, we can assume that their spouses are even more in the dark."*

That sounds like a challenge. Now that you've read *Your Guy's Guide to Gynecology*, you're ready to prove how wrong this assumption can be—and just how much of a positive impact you can have during a difficult time in your partner's life.

We believe that *you* will be the best person to determine what your partner needs if you make the effort. Even if you remember little of what you've read, patience, consistency, and caring will lead you down the right road.

Women in the following situations may have a particularly difficult time adjusting to hysterectomy (but remember that *any* woman can have trouble)**:

- premenopausal women;
- women who didn't have children;
- women with little formal education, especially education about human anatomy;
- women with previous psychiatric problems (particularly those with a history of molestation or abuse);
- women showing particularly high levels of depression or anxiety before surgery;
- women who have emergency hysterectomy, leaving them no time to prepare;
- women with cancer, especially if radical (more extensive) surgery is needed;
- women without a significant relationship before the operation.

Returning to Full Activity

Expect to wait six to eight weeks after surgery for healing to take place. Do not "push the envelope" on this healing time; a too-early return to exercise or intercourse may cause her severe pain and serious injury.

*R. Stellman, *Gynecology and Obstetrics*, 6. ed., Sciarra, chapter 90. Philadelphia: Lippincott, 1999.
**M. Hollender, "A study of patients admitted to a psychiatric hospital after pelvic operations," *American Journal of Obstetrics and Gynecology* 79(3): 489 (1960). Although this is an older study, we believe its conclusions are still valid.

After a major operation, it is natural for you both to be a little anxious when you begin your physical relationship again. It helps to be patient and let her control the pace as much as you can. She may initially have some discomfort with intercourse. If she controls the insertion of your penis and the positions you use, she is likely to be more relaxed. Lubricants are a good idea; they can be obtained from a drugstore without a prescription. As she begins to feel confident again with her body, her own lubrication should increase.

 Don't be surprised if your sex life improves! After an operation that removes a source of pelvic pain and/or chronic bleeding, many women feel liberated.

A recent prospective study of more than 1,200 women in Maryland examined their sexual function before and after hysterectomy. Sex drive and frequency of intercourse all increased, and pain with intercourse decreased after surgery.*

There may be some challenges for your relationship after hysterectomy. As mentioned, the emotional reaction to hysterectomy may take some time to surface and be resolved. Physical problems can occur as well. Healing may be prolonged, perhaps because of infection or complications of surgery.

If her ovaries were removed and she had not yet reached the menopause, she will experience a rapid fall in estrogen levels. This may cause no symptoms at all, or she may be plagued with mood swings, insomnia, hot flashes, and vaginal dryness. Treatment with estrogen replacement will usually relieve these symptoms. Patience is a virtue, as the dose of estrogen may need to be adjusted. Lubricants often help with vaginal dryness as well.

A small minority of women seem to experience a loss of interest in sex after hysterectomy. This is often temporary and improves over time, as the healing process completes itself. Occasionally, women suffer a more prolonged loss of interest caused by a change in their body sensations with intercourse. They may find their orgasm has diminished in intensity due to the removal of the uterus (it contracts strongly with orgasm).

*G. M. Guzinski et al., "Hysterectomy and sexual functioning," *Journal of the American Medical Association* 282: 1934–1941 (1999).

Another theory relates a loss of sex drive after hysterectomy to the removal of the *ovaries*, which make a small amount of testosterone (the male hormone). Testosterone replacement in women is an area of active research, but not much is known with certainty at this time. Low-dose testosterone can be tried in select cases if no other approach is helpful. Testosterone does have side effects, including enlargement of the clitoris, hair growth, and possible liver damage, so care must be taken in using this potent hormone.

The answer to the problem of sexual difficulties following hysterectomy may be simple or complex. Issues relating to the surgery itself, her emotional reaction to it, and the dynamics of your relationship may need to be addressed. If the problems don't seem to be getting better despite your best efforts, the two of you should speak to her doctor. It's important not to wait too long to seek help. Communication is a key element in resolving these kinds of problems; see Supportive Guy's recommendations on page 220 for suggestions.

In Conclusion

Hysterectomy is a common surgery, although the many new treatment options available are already decreasing its use. The vast majority of women undergoing this operation recover fully and go on to live healthier, happier lives.

Your partner's decision to have a hysterectomy is a major one, and your participation is important. Congratulations on your decision to play an active and informed role in your partner's life. The results of your efforts will be with both of you for years to come.

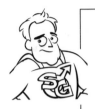

Supportive Guy's Recommendations If Your Partner Needs Surgery

1. Talk with her about her problem. She'll feel better if you know what she's going through and what she's doing about it. This is perhaps the most important thing that you can do, and it should go on throughout the course of her problem. Ask questions, and really listen to her answers.

2. Make sure that both of you understand the proposed treatments, alternatives, and risks involved. *Your Guy's Guide to Gynecology* may answer some of your questions. Encourage her to speak again with her doctor if she's confused or worried about her treatment.

3. If she's having a hysterectomy, learn as much as you can about what to expect before the operation. Many centers offer prehysterectomy workshops for both partners—a great source of information.

4. Help her to comply with activity restrictions. Before surgery, she may not be able to exercise or enjoy intercourse. Once she comes home after an operation, she should receive detailed instructions about activity, diet, and danger signs. It may be some time before she can get back to strenuous activity. Don't rush the process; the consequences can be severe.

5. If possible, take her to the hospital for surgery yourself. Speak to her doctor after surgery. She'll be recovering, so you will probably be the best person for her doctor to give specific information to. When she's more awake and relaxed, you can share with her the details of her operation.

6. Help out more around the house while she's recovering so she can relax.

7. Help her remember to take her medicines. Most of us aren't used to taking medications. If she's been prescribed something for pain, anemia, or to control her bleeding, help her remember to take it.

(continued)

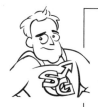

8. After surgery, watch for the danger signs. If she has heavy bleeding, dizziness, persistent nausea and vomiting, or an elevated temperature she may need urgent care.

9. Encourage follow-up visits. She will need to speak with her doctor to confirm the findings at surgery and make a long-range plan for follow-up.

10. If she has lost a pregnancy, be alert for signs of grieving. Encourage her to talk about her sadness, and to cry when she needs to. Don't feel funny if you need to cry, too. This process may take several weeks. If either of you seems to be having a particularly hard time, contact her doctor. There are support groups in most communities for couples dealing with pregnancy loss.

POST TEST

1. Hysteroscopy is performed along with a D & C to improve the diagnostic and therapeutic outcomes of the procedure.
   T or F

2. A D & C can be used to control abnormal bleeding from the uterus that doesn't respond to medical treatment.
   T or F

3. Most simple ovarian cysts will require surgery.
   T or F

4. Severe lower abdominal pain requiring emergency surgery may be a result of an ovarian cyst.
   T or F

5. Tubal pregnancies may be successfully treated without surgery.
   T or F

6. The chance of having another tubal pregnancy goes down after the first occurrence.
   T or F

7. Laparoscopic surgery has all but replaced open surgery for ectopic pregnancies.
   T or F

8. After hysterectomy, menstrual bleeding typically increases for a few months.
   T or F

9. Loss of sex drive is uncommon after hysterectomy.
   T or F

10. A Supportive Guy would be present for prehysterectomy appointments with his partner's doctor and would play an active role in decision-making and emotional support.
    T or F

Key: 1.T 2.T 3.F 4.T 5.T 6.F 7.T 8.F 9.T 10. True!

SO, YOU WANT TO HAVE A BABY 9

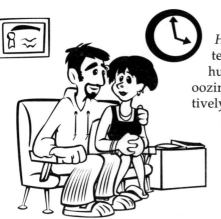

B oy, this is it! The official entrance to the Great State of Adulthood: *Having a baby!* Just think about it—centering your life around a newborn human child: a screaming, crying, oozing, rapidly dividing mass of primitively connected neurons that hardly knows what it wants from moment to moment: a little creature that will quickly make *your* desires only a distant memory.

You thought you gave up everything just to have a relationship! But seriously now, a baby? A BABY?? How did you get talked into this? Because you're in love, she's "the right one," and you've both contracted a bad case of Perfect Baby Syndrome! This common disorder affects men as well as women and is responsible for countless victims of the current baby boom. Simply put, persons with this condition think they're going to have a Perfect Baby.

Perfect Babies, it is believed, are always cute and cuddly; they coo on request and play quietly in their cribs when not needed. These babies are also dry, having virtually no tendency to leak fluids from body cavities on themselves or on anyone else who might be nearby.

These miraculous creatures are also good sleepers. They look forward to bedtime, falling peacefully asleep at precisely ten minutes before the start of *Ally McBeal* or other desired prime-time programming. Their body clocks awaken them consistently at 7:00 A.M., or 8:30 on the weekends.

Finally, Perfect Babies are considerate. They are careful not to disrupt normal routines, including but not limited to eating, showering, car-washing, and especially the very type of horizontal activity that begat the Perfect Baby to begin with.

People afflicted with Perfect Baby Syndrome cling desperately to the belief that these creatures actually exist, not unlike the Tooth Fairy, Santa Claus, and the Balanced Budget. No amount of education, advice, or therapy can deter those afflicted from the anticipated arrival of their blessed bundle.

Since there is no cure for Perfect Baby Syndrome, the best we can offer is advice on how to have a *healthy* pregnancy. In this, the final chapter of *Your Guy's Guide to Gynecology*, we provide answers to the most commonly asked questions couples have before conception. Read on, and then proceed with caution. And don't say we didn't warn you.

GUY-Q TEST

1. Pre-pregnancy diets should include which of the following?
   a. Folic acid
   b. Caffeine
   c. Saint-John's-wort
   d. All of the above

2. Diabetic women should prepare for pregnancy by:
   a. decreasing their insulin dose.
   b. increasing their starch intake.
   c. carefully controlling their blood sugar.
   d. all of the above.

3. Which of these medical conditions can adversely affect pregnancy?
   a. Diabetes
   b. High blood pressure
   c. Lupus
   d. Chronic kidney disease
   e. All of the above

4. Which of these drugs may harm a developing baby?
   a. Vitamin C
   b. Antiseizure medications
   c. Laxatives
   d. Isotretinoin
   e. b and d only

5. Maternal age over 35 is associated with:
   a. fewer miscarriages.
   b. babies with higher IQs.
   c. a lower rate of cesarean section.
   d. a greater chance of chromosomal problems in the baby.

6. Which of the following is a sign of ovulation?
   a. The start of menstrual flow
   b. A brief sharp pain in the lower abdomen
   c. Headaches and water retention
   d. Decreased sex drive

7. Cigarette smoking increases the chances of:
   a. miscarriage.
   b. growth restriction of the fetus.
   c. placental problems.
   d. preterm delivery.
   e. sudden infant death syndrome.
   f. all of the above.

8. The most critical time in fetal development to avoid drug exposure is:
   a. the first trimester.
   b. the second trimester.
   c. the third trimester.

9. Chemicals found in some workplaces that may cause problems in pregnancy include:
   a. asbestos.
   b. detergents.
   c. air fresheners.
   d. organic solvents.

10. You can improve your chances of conceiving a baby by:
    a. having sex only when she's having a period.
    b. having sex at least twice a day all month long.
    c. having sex at ovulation after abstaining from sex for two days.
    d. eating oysters, watching football, and then having sex.

Key: 1. a 2. c 3. e 4. e 5. d 6. b 7. f 8. a 9. d 10. c

PRECONCEPTION COUNSELING

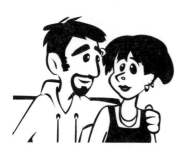

A healthy new trend in obstetrics is the preconception counseling appointment. At this visit, a couple can learn about important changes in diet, medication, or lifestyle that should be made before getting pregnant. Testing of either prospective parent may be needed to prevent problems. A healthy outcome for both mother and baby is more likely with this kind of planning.

What Should She Eat?

We recommend that your partner eat a well-balanced, healthy diet before and during her pregnancy. The average woman needs approximately 2,200 calories per day; when she becomes pregnant, she will need an additional 300 calories per day.

Women who are vegetarians may need minor changes in their diet to provide for healthy development of a baby. It's a very good idea for vegetarians or anyone with an unusual diet to see a nutritionist before becoming pregnant.

Eating raw meat is not wise for a woman considering pregnancy because of the possibility of acquiring toxoplasmosis. This parasitic infection can cause serious problems for a newborn, including hydrocephalus and mental retardation. This infection can also be acquired by handling cat feces, so someone else should change the litter box (hint) during pregnancy.

Pregnant women should stay away from unpasteurized milk, soft cheese, undercooked hot dogs or chicken, and unwashed fruit or vegetables. Eating these foods can increase the risk of infection from listeria, a bacteria that can cause abortion, stillbirth, or preterm labor.

Also, research has shown that consumption of excessive amounts of coffee (more than three cups per day, in one study) raised the chances of miscarriage. The risks of premature labor, birth defects, and growth retardation may be increased as well. Although an occasional cup of coffee or tea is probably safe, it's best to quit or cut back on caffeine consumption before pregnancy.

Some recent studies have focused on zinc deficiency and its impact on pregnancy. In a Scandinavian study, women with low serum zinc levels had a higher rate of babies born with birth defects. Other studies suggest that deficient zinc intake may raise the chances of premature birth and low birth weight. Zinc is typically found in animal proteins; therefore, vegetarians may not be getting enough zinc from their diet.

S. Jameson, "Effects of zinc deficiency in human reproduction," *Acta Med Scandanavia* supplement: 593–600 (1976).

In addition to specific dietary habits, a woman's body weight is important to consider before pregnancy. Problem pregnancies are more common in women who are either very overweight or underweight before pregnancy. Specifically, obese women have a greater risk of complications like gestational (pregnancy-induced) diabetes and high blood pressure, birth injuries, cesarean sections, and postdelivery problems. Underweight women are prone to give birth to babies who are growth restricted (malnourished). Weight problems are best corrected before pregnancy is attempted.

Important note: it is best to avoid diet pills and all unecessary medications when attempting conception! Many drugs have the potential to harm the fetus before a woman realizes she's pregnant.

Should She Take Vitamins?

For a woman planning a pregnancy, a healthy diet and the avoidance of smoking, drugs, and alcohol are far more important than taking vitamins.

One important exception to this is folic acid. Research has shown that taking folic acid before and during pregnancy lowers the risk of having a child with neural tube defects (NTDs) like spina bifida. NTDs are the most common major birth defects.

The U.S. Public Health Service currently recommends that all women planning pregnancy supplement their diet with 0.4 milligrams of folate per day. A woman who has already had a child with an NTD must take 4.0 milligrams of folate per day to lower her risk of having another affected child.

Many multivitamins contain folic acid. It also can be found in leafy, dark green vegetables, citrus fruits, beans, bread, and fortified cereals.

Folate must be started *before conception* and continued through the first trimester of pregnancy for it to be effective in lowering the risk of neural tube defects.

Care must be taken in the use of vitamin supplements. For example, high-dose vitamin A intake during pregnancy has been associated with growth restriction and birth defects in newborns. Apparently, the amount required for these adverse effects is commonly found in many multivitamin preparations. *Prenatal* vitamins typically contain safe doses of vitamin A. Women should review their vitamin supplements with an obstetrician before attempting pregnancy.

At the present time, we don't have enough evidence to conclude that the popular herbal remedies echinacea and Saint-John's-wort can be safely used during pregnancy.

Does She Need Any Special Tests Before Pregnancy?

Her doctor will probably recommend testing for immunity to rubella. Rubella (German measles) can cause severe birth defects if acquired during pregnancy. If immunity is absent, it is common practice to immunize the woman and ask her to wait for three months (for the immunity to take effect) before conceiving.

Testing for immunity to hepatitis B is also a good idea for any woman at increased risk for this disease. Health care workers, lab personnel exposed to blood or blood products, and people from areas of the world where hepatitis B is common (for example, southeast Asia) are at greatest risk. The hepatitis B vaccine can be given during pregnancy, but it makes more sense to give it before conception and protect both the fetus and mother.

Infants born to women with hepatitis B often become chronic carriers of the infection. Not only can they infect others, they can suffer chronic liver damage from the infection. According to an article in the medical journal *Lancet*, 25% of chronic carriers of hepatitis B will eventually die from liver-related disease.*

Chicken pox (varicella) testing is also recommended before conception. If acquired during pregnancy, this common childhood infection may cause birth defects or severe infection in the newborn. For those without immunity to chicken pox, vaccination is recommended before conception, with a three-month waiting period following.

Testing for anemia (low blood count) may allow for correction of the deficiency with oral iron tablets before pregnancy. Women who are anemic will be more fatigued during their pregnancy and may be more susceptible to illness. In addition, delivery will more likely result in a need for a blood transfusion if a woman is significantly anemic before giving birth.

Certain types of anemia are inherited as problems with the red blood cell itself; they cannot be cured with iron supplementation. These anemias are important because they may complicate pregnancy and also may be passed on to the newborn, sometimes with catastrophic results. Sickle-cell disease is caused by an abnormal hemoglobin molecule, which impairs the red blood cell's ability to carry oxygen. All African American women should be screened for this disease if they are anemic. All women of Mediterranean, southeast Asian, and African American descent also need testing for another red cell disorder, thalassemia. Partners of these women may need testing as well, to see if they, too, have abnormal red blood cells.

Another test that may be ordered before pregnancy is one to detect Tay-Sachs disease. When one or both partners is of Ashkenazi Jewish, Cajun, or French Canadian descent, or when there is a history of Tay-Sachs disease in the family, this blood test is necessary. Tay-Sachs disease is caused by the deficiency of a particular enzyme, which leads to the accumulation of a chemical within cells. This may sound harmless, but the effects of Tay-Sachs are disastrous for the young who inherit it: mental retardation, seizures, and blindness. Early diagnosis allows for couples to be counseled about the risks of transmitting this disease to their child during pregnancy.

---

*R. P. Beasly et al., "Prevention of perinatally transmitted hepatitis B virus infections with hepatitis B immune globulin and hepatitis vaccine," *Lancet* 2: 1099–1102 (1983).

In general, it's a good idea to consult with an obstetrician or genetics specialist if a close family member has a significant birth defect or mental retardation.

An obstetrician may also recommend testing for sexually transmitted diseases. Chlamydia, gonorrhea, genital herpes, and syphilis can all cause significant problems during pregnancy (for more information on STDs, see Chapter 4). Chlamydia, gonorrhea, and syphilis can be cured when diagnosed before pregnancy begins. Although we don't yet have a cure for herpes, the diagnosis is valuable because steps can be taken to protect the fetus from acquiring the infection.

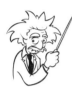

Another STD of great importance is AIDS (for more information, see Chapter 5). Studies have shown that a high percentage (25–40%) of pregnant women with the HIV virus will pass it to their children.* Treatment with AZT during pregnancy will substantially lower that risk. This makes an early HIV test an excellent idea for all women contemplating pregnancy.

*M. Gwinn et al., "Prevalence of HIV infection in childbearing women in the U.S.: Surveillance using newborn blood samples," *Journal of the American Medical Association* 265: 1704 (1991).

Another test of significance before pregnancy is a skin test for tuberculosis. Health care workers, women from areas where tuberculosis is common, or those living with someone who has had the disease should be tested.

What If She Has Medical Problems and Wants to Get Pregnant?

For specific information on an illness and how it affects pregnancy, as well as how pregnancy may alter the disease itself, it's best to consult an obstetrician. Here we will briefly mention a few of the more common conditions and their impact on pregnancy.

Women with insulin-dependent diabetes have been shown to have babies with major birth defects three times more often than the general population. The good news is that there is now strong evidence that careful control of blood sugar *before conception* and through the first three months of pregnancy will significantly lower that risk.

Tight control of blood sugars before conception is crucial for any diabetic woman considering pregnancy.

In addition, diabetic women often give birth to large (macrosomic) babies. These babies are more likely to require cesarean section or to suffer birth injuries during vaginal delivery. Good control of blood sugar and close cooperation with a doctor can lower these risks.

Finally, certain advanced stages of diabetes may carry such high risks for the mother that pregnancy may not be a good idea at all. If your partner has had diabetes for a long time and has significant kidney disease or high blood pressure, you both should talk to her doctor before planning a pregnancy.

Another common medical condition, hypertension (high blood pressure), may cause problems for pregnant women. Women with hypertension are more likely to have problems with premature delivery, stillbirth, toxemia, and fetal growth restriction.

Not all hypertension treatments are safe for pregnancy, either. One class of medications, angiotensin-converting-enzyme inhibitors, can cause birth defects and stillbirths. If your partner has high blood pressure, she should consult her doctor before pregnancy to make sure that she is on the best medicine and the right dose.

Pregnancies complicated by seizure disorders have a greater risk of complications. Babies born to mothers who suffer from seizures have a higher rate of birth defects, growth restriction in utero, and developmental delay. Unfortunately, many medications given to control seizures have the potential for fetal harm as well. Valproic acid and carbamazepine may cause neural tube defects, and amniocentesis may be needed to detect this problem if one of these medications must be used. Overall, most women with seizure disorders will have healthy babies, but it is vital that a woman with this problem see her doctor before conceiving.

Many other illnesses will be complicated by pregnancy or can cause problems for the fetus. Any woman with asthma, thyroid disease, systemic lupus erythematosus (SLE), heart or kidney disease, phenylketonuria, a history of blood clots, cancer, or other serious conditions should see an obstetrician before conception.

A few illnesses are so dangerous in pregnancy that a woman should be discouraged from having children altogether. Some of these conditions are primary pulmonary hypertension, advanced diabetes, severe cardiac disease, and moderate or severe kidney failure.

When Should She Stop Smoking/Taking Drugs/Consuming Alcohol?

Once conception occurs, the major organs of the baby begin to form within a few days. The heart, the kidneys, the liver, literally all of the person-to-be is established by eight weeks after conception. Many women aren't even aware they're pregnant until then. So, taking drugs, smoking, or drinking alcohol now can lead to a miscarriage or major problems for the baby when it's born. If either of you smokes, takes drugs, or abuses alcohol, quit now, before you conceive.

Cigarette smoking increases the risk of miscarriage, growth restriction in utero (in the womb), premature rupture of the membranes, premature delivery, and placental problems, all increasing the risk of fetal death. Some studies say smoking in pregnancy lowers intelligence in offspring. After birth, smoking cigarettes in the household contributes to crib death (sudden infant death syndrome), bronchitis, and chronic lung disease in children.

This is, of course, presuming you and/or your partner don't care about the chronic lung conditions like emphysema you're likely to get from smoking, the premature aging and wrinkling of the skin, the smelly clothes and breath, and the significant risk of dying prematurely and miserably from bladder, throat, or lung cancer. Here's a message for your partner: more women die these days from lung cancer (thanks to smoking) than from breast cancer.

Drugs? Remember those commercials showing the egg frying in the pan, "This is your brain on drugs"? Well, apply that same analogy to the poor fetus that's trying to develop while drugs are being pumped into him or her through the placenta. Here's a few more specifics:

Marijuana increases premature labor, growth restriction in utero, and seems to cause behavior changes in newborns. Cocaine is well known to cause an obstetric emergency called placental abruption. This means that the placenta, which is the fetus's only oxygen and nutrition supply, suddenly shears away from the wall of the uterus. Placental abruption often leads to rapid and irreversible oxygen deprivation and fetal death; a fetus that survives a placental abruption may be born with severe brain damage. Evidence is also accumulating that cocaine causes birth defects. Intravenous narcotics like heroin are linked to poor fetal growth, and acquiring HIV is a risk of heroin use, because of needle sharing among addicts.

A socially acceptable drug that can also be extremely harmful to a pregnancy is alcohol. Although an occasional (rare) glass of wine is probably harmless, moderate to heavy drinking while pregnant is associated with an increased risk of miscarriage as well as a pattern of abnormalities in the baby, known as fetal alcohol syndrome. According to one authoritative text, the major features of this preventable condition include growth restriction, a deformed face, mental retardation, and heart defects.

If you need help stopping drug or alcohol use or smoking, get it! Feeling guilty without changing your behavior won't help you or your children. Your doctor would be thrilled to direct you to a program that works for you.

One of the great things about planning to have a family is that it's an excellent excuse to start living in a way that supports your *own* life and health as well as your child's.

Should She Stop Her Medications?

Most medicines, either prescribed or over-the-counter, are probably not harmful in pregnancy. On the flip side, most medications have been incompletely studied in pregnancy, and it's often difficult to be absolutely sure they are free from risk.

Therefore, it's become standard to urge women contemplating pregnancy to discontinue any unnecessary drugs before conceiving a child. The key is to decide which medicines aren't necessary; this is best done in consultation with a doctor.

The rate of major birth defects is 3 to 4 per 100 births in the United States. This means that every couple attempting to have a child has about a 3½ percent risk of having a child with a birth defect (some conditions, like maternal diabetes, increase the risk of birth defects). Stopping unnecessary medications, especially if their risk is unknown, may improve the chances of having a healthy baby.

The following are some of the drugs believed to be harmful to a developing fetus, if taken during pregnancy:

- phenytoin, carbamazepine, valproic acid, and trimethadione (antiseizure medications);
- aminopterin and methotrexate (anticancer drugs);
- isotretinoin (treatment for acne);
- warfarin (anticoagulant);
- lithium (treatment for certain psychiatric disorders);
- tetracycline (antibiotic);
- angiotensin-converting-enzyme inhibitors (new class of antihypertension medications).

Medical conditions that need treatment can often be managed with safer medications during pregnancy. Talk to her doctor about this.

When Should She Stop Her Birth Control Pills?

Up until recently, there was a lot of concern about the possibility of fetal harm from oral contraceptives. This led to a recommendation to stop taking the pill a few months before conception was attempted. We have learned, however, that birth control pills have no harmful effects on the fetus, even if they are inadvertently taken for the first eight weeks of pregnancy.

One circumstance that might prompt us to recommend stopping the pill long before conception is when a woman is planning a pregnancy during her later reproductive years (after age 35). Studies show that women *may* not conceive as quickly for the first year after oral contraceptives are stopped. Although there is no permanent effect on fertility, this temporary decrease wouldn't be the best thing for a woman who doesn't have much time.

The other common forms of hormonal contraception, Depo-Provera injections and Norplant, also do not require a waiting period after discontinuation before starting a family. Norplant, the long-acting progesterone capsule, has the added advantage of a prompt return to normal fertility rates as soon as the capsules are removed. Because it inhibits ovulation, Depo-Provera may temporarily reduce fertility, as birth control pills do.

Another contraceptive chemical that has raised concern about possible fetal harm is nonoxynol-9. This spermicide, often used with condoms and diaphragms, has never been shown to have adverse effects on pregnancies. Therefore, couples may continue to use barrier methods with nonoxynol-9 even if they think she may have already conceived.

What if There's a History of Pregnancy Problems in Her Family or Mine?

Miscarriage is a far more common event than most couples realize. Learning that the women in either family suffered a miscarriage during their reproductive life is usually not a sign of a true reproductive problem.

Statistics tell us that at least 15 to 20% of pregnancies miscarry; the number would probably go a lot higher if we detected all conceptions that occur.

However, any couple with a family history of *frequent* unexplained pregnancy loss or birth defects should make sure to see her obstetrician before pregnancy.

If either family has a history of genetic disorders like Tay-Sachs disease, Fragile X syndrome, Down's syndrome, sickle-cell anemia, thalassemia, or cystic fibrosis, preconception counseling is a must. The same holds true if either member of a couple is known to be a carrier of any genetic disorder. *Before* pregnancy is the best time to discuss potential risks.

Most reproductive problems are *not* passed on to succeeding generations. However, certain illnesses like diabetes and sickle-cell disease, if inherited by the mother-to-be, can lead to complications of pregnancy. As mentioned above, significant health problems such as these should be discussed with her doctor before conception.

What if She's Had Problems in a Prior Pregnancy?

Most pregnancy complications are minor and won't recur in future pregnancies. Others can be prevented or successfully managed during the pregnancy itself and don't require advance planning. The exceptions that might really suggest a preconception visit to her obstetrician would be:

- if she's had two or more spontaneous abortions (miscarriages) and no live births;
- if she's been told she has an incompetent (weakened) cervix;
- if she was exposed to DES (an estrogenic medication) while in utero (her mother took the medicine during pregnancy);
- if she's given birth to a previous child with a birth defect;
- if she's had an ectopic pregnancy;
- if she's had a prior stillborn child;
- if she's delivered a child more than three weeks before her due date.

Does My Job (or Hers) Affect Our Chances for Having a Healthy Child?

The vast majority of work environments are safe for couples considering pregnancy. Rarely, a particular job causes enough exposure to harmful chemicals that the chance of miscarriage and/or birth defects is increased. Employers are required by law to inform you of these risks.

Examples of chemicals found in some workplaces that may be hazardous to future fertility (they can damage sperm!) include organic solvents, vinyl monomers, chemicals used in photography, pesticides, and heavy metals like lead or mercury. Health care workers should avoid prolonged exposures to anticancer drugs, radiation, and anesthetic gases.

If you have any questions about either of your work exposures, talk to your employers and to her doctor.

A more common issue has to do with the incompatibility of pregnancy and a physically demanding job. Some women may not be able to continue this type of job throughout pregnancy. Nightshift work or a job that requires lifting bulky or heavy objects is not usually recommended. You might want to discuss these issues with your doctor in advance.

What if I'm (or She's) Older?

"Older" in reproductive terms for a woman starts around the age of 35. Of course, women at 35 are not really old; it's just that the number of years of future fertility at that age is somewhat limited. In addition, the risk of certain reproductive problems increases beyond that age. For example:

- Becoming pregnant may be more difficult because fertility rates begin to decline in her 30s.

- The rate of chromosomal problems like Down's syndrome at the age of 35 is about one in 200, or 0.5%. The odds of having a chromosomally abnormal infant increase gradually from there, and are more than one percent by the age of 40 (rates increase more rapidly after that). Amniocentesis and chorionic villus sampling are two tests that check the chromosomes of a developing fetus in the first half of pregnancy.

- The rate of spontaneous miscarriage increases with age.

- Women over 35 have a slightly greater chance of giving birth to fraternal (nonidentical) twins. Multiple pregnancies are high-risk at any age.

- Women over 35 have more chronic medical conditions. Specifically, they have a higher incidence of gestational (pregnancy-induced) diabetes and hypertension.

- For reasons that are still unclear, babies born to "older" women are more likely to need to be delivered by cesarean section.

Fathers-to-be contribute just as much to the chromosomal makeup of their new baby. Current information suggests that sperm don't become abnormal in the same way as eggs can before conception, but sperm may have spontaneous mutations that cause problems in their offspring. The age at which mutations seem to increase is around 35.

The number of women giving birth later in life has risen dramatically in the past 20 years. Although there are some risks, most women who become pregnant at 35 or older have normal pregnancies and deliver healthy children.

How Can We Make It Happen (Sooner)?

The miraculous microscopic event of conception evades our full understanding and certainly our attempts at controlling it. Even when couples are willing to submit to the wondrous maneuvers practiced by fertility specialists, the results are sometimes unexpected or undesired. Therefore, the whole idea of "making it happen" when referring to a pregnancy must be understood to be, at best, optimistic. So, what's an eager couple to do?

First, since you've read Chapter 1, you know when your partner's fertile time is. The idea then is quite simple: you should make love around the time of ovulation. How do you do that?

Ovulation can be detected at home by the following methods:

- If your partner has regular menstrual cycles, count back 14 days from the first day of her period; a woman with a 30-day cycle would be ovulating on day 16 (for a 28-day cycle, day 14, etc.).

- Watch for the physical signs of ovulation. Most women will note some vague lower abdominal pain and an increase in their discharge around ovulation. The presence of these symptoms suggests ovulation may have occurred, but it may certainly happen without them, too.

- Use a basal body thermometer (BBT). This special thermometer, when properly used, can detect the subtle increase in body temperature that occurs with ovulation (and lasts until her period—unless she becomes pregnant). BBTs can be purchased at most pharmacies, but beware—they must be used exactly as specified.

- Use an ovulation predictor kit. Remember from Figure 1.3 of Chapter 1 that a woman's luteinizing hormone (LH) rises just before ovulation. Ovulation predictor kits enable women to test their urine to detect that LH surge. These kits are widely available at pharmacies and drugstores.

You maximize your chances of getting pregnant by making love every other day, starting about 3 or 4 days before ovulation is expected. Continue this until a few days after she ovulates. We also advise against douching during this time and recommend the woman lie quietly for at least an hour after sex.

 We then remind couples that even if they do everything right, it may take more than a year to conceive.

When Should We See an Infertility Specialist?

For most couples, we advise seeing an infertility specialist after a year of attempting pregnancy without success. We also tell them that it's likely that nothing is wrong and they just need a little more time.

For couples with problems known to cause infertility, we make the referral sooner. Examples would be women with significant ovulation disorders, blocked fallopian tubes, or prior infertility, or men with sperm problems. We also might refer a couple earlier if the woman is 40 years of age or older.

When Should We Begin Prenatal Care?

We like to see our obstetric patients (and their partners) at six to ten weeks after her last menstrual period. This allows adequate time to assess the health of the mother and the pregnancy. It's also a good time to begin educating the couple about how to take care of themselves during their pregnancy.

POST TEST

1. Pregnant women need an extra 5,000 calories a day to provide for the baby's needs.
   T or F

2. Vitamin A is helpful in pregnancy, and the more the better.
   T or F

3. A newborn with "fetal alcohol syndrome" will have a high blood alcohol level at birth.
   T or F

4. Diabetic women should maintain close control of blood sugars before and after conception.
   T or F

5. High blood pressure has no effect on pregnancy.
   T or F

6. Birth control pills should be stopped three months before conception.
   T or F

7. The odds of a chromosomal problem increase with maternal age.
   T or F

8. Fetal problems may be increased with the *father's* age.
   T or F

9. Infertility is the inability to achieve pregnancy within one year with the same partner and using timed intercourse.
   T or F

10. Perfect Babies are always cute and cuddly.
    T or F

Key: 1. F   2. F   3. F   4. T   5. F   6. F   7. T   8. T   9. T
        10. True, but there's no such thing as a Perfect Baby!

ADDENDUM: THE PELVIC EXAM

An office visit to a gynecologist will vary widely in content and style, depending on the training and personality of the doctor, as well as the purpose of the visit. This chapter summarizes only the most common and important parts of the typical visit, so that you as a male can understand why your partner looks at you and says, "You're lucky *you* don't have to go."

The nurse checks the patient in: "Hello, Mrs. Pearl. Before the doctor sees you, I'd like to check your blood pressure and your weight. What brings you to see the doctor today?"

(The patient replies.)

The nurse summarizes the patient's response in writing for the doctor, and then says:

"We'd like you to put on this paper gown. The doctor will be with you shortly."

The patient is left alone in the room to change into the gown, and then to wonder why, with so many people there dressed only in paper gowns, the thermostat is set at 65 degrees.

The doctor enters, greets the patient, and begins to interview her with general, open-ended questions: "Good afternoon, Mrs. Pearl. I understand you're having some trouble with your menstrual periods. What can you tell me about that?"

The questions become more specific in order to define the problem:

"When did the problem start? How many days of bleeding did you have? Do you have cramps as well?"

Since quite often patients do not bring up difficult issues at the beginning of a visit, a good technique is to ask once again, "Was there anything else you wanted to talk about?"

What Other Questions Might a Gynecologist Ask?

Once the physician is convinced he or she has obtained enough information about the patient's major concerns, he or she will ask about the patient's past medical and surgical history, current medications, social situation, habits (smoking, alcohol, and drug use), and pertinent family history. Then it's time to proceed to the physical examination.

How Is the Physical Exam Done?

These days, the gynecologist is often recognized as a primary care physician, expanding the range of his or her clinical duties to diagnosis and treatment of more general conditions, such as hypertension or thyroid disease. For the purposes of this book, however, we have elected to include only those parts of the exam that are specific to gynecology.

Exam of the Breasts

A thorough visual and tactile inspection of the breasts and surrounding tissues is made to detect lumps (masses), enlarged lymph nodes, nipple discharge, and even subtle skin changes that might indicate an early cancer.

Exam of the Abdomen

The abdomen is carefully inspected to detect tenderness and/or to identify enlarged organs (liver, spleen, or a pelvic mass arising from the uterus or an ovary). Surgical scars on the abdomen are matched to the patient's surgical history.

Exam of the Pelvis

The pelvic exam is broken down into two distinct parts:

- **External genitalia** With the patient lying on her back, her feet are placed in stirrups. Then she moves her buttocks forward to the very edge of the examining table. The vulva is inspected for discharge or abnormal tissue that may indicate infection, chronic irritative conditions, or early signs of cancer. Anatomic structures such as the labia minora and majora and the Bartholin's glands are examined.

The vagina and cervix are inspected using an instrument known as a speculum (see Figure A.1), which allows easy visualization of these surfaces. Their appearance is noted, along with an assessment of what is known as pelvic support. Childbirth or middle age may result in a loss of this support, causing the bladder, uterus, intestines, or rectum to protrude into the vagina. With the speculum in place, a Pap smear of the cervix may be obtained. As is explained in Chapter 7, this test requires a gentle scraping of the cervix to obtain cells for microscopic exam. Excessive or abnormal-appearing vaginal or cervical fluid (discharge) can be sampled for culture or examined under a microscope to detect infection. The speculum is then removed.

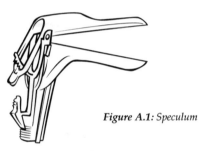

Figure A.1: *Speculum*

- **Internal or bimanual exam**   With the patient in the same position on the table, the examiner then uses both hands to feel the uterus and attached, or adnexal, structures, the ovaries and tubes. The doctor will use the second and third fingers of one (gloved) hand in the vagina to lift these organs up and then feel them by pressing down on the abdominal wall above them with the other hand. The size, position, consistency (hard or soft), and mobility of both the uterus and the ovaries are assessed. The space beneath the uterus, appropriately named the cul-de-sac, is checked, because an enlarged ovary may sometimes be found there. In addition, the cul-de-sac is a frequent site for a disease known as endometriosis (see Chapter 7). The bimanual exam may be supplemented by placing an additional finger into the rectum; then it, too, can be assessed for tumors or abnormalities, as well as provide additional information about the status of the cul-de-sac.

At this point, the pelvic exam is complete. Once the woman has had a moment to dress, the findings and plan for her care can be discussed.

Aren't you glad you'll never need a Pap smear?

ACKNOWLEDGMENTS

Book writing is an unfamiliar task to the two of us, having done little other than running around hospitals and clinics, caring for patients, for the past twenty (!) years. Whatever writing we did previously was typically brief and predictably illegible.

Many people were instrumental in helping us translate our raw inspiration, to teach men about women's bodies, into the printed pages that follow. Without their energy, faith, and patience, a book such as this would never have materialized.

First and foremost, to David Brake, whose belief in our basic idea and long-term attention to its development kept us going and shaped the book itself. To Richard Louv, a fine writer for the *San Diego Union Tribune*, who gave us the name for this book one evening over a glass of wine at his home. To John Ready, an attorney and friend, who provided enthusiastic support while translating the legalese of partnership contracts. To the following OB/GYN physicians, who provided their clinical expertise and encouragement: Charles March, Robert Israel, Paul Brenner, and Dan Mishell of Women's Hospital at L.A. County-U.S.C. Medical Center; Jane Bening, Stuart Fischbein, Charles Nager of the U.C. San Diego Department of Reproductive Medicine; and our partners at Kaiser Permanente in San Diego, Clement Hoffman, David Preskill, Karl Luber, Paul Koonings, James Price, Michael Manley, Leslie Casper-Moberg, and Joseph Fremont.

To Epazote's restaurant, located near the ocean in the village of Del Mar, whose awe-inspiring view was the inspiration we needed in the early days of this project.

To our "San Diego team" that actually put the book together: Cyndi Hawkes made pages and helped coordinate, Nichole Smith provided brilliant cover designs, Lynn Harris somehow edited the raw material, and Steve Troop drew our characters and discovered he could even do medical illustrations.

To the guys that attend the men's class each month at Kaiser Hospital in San Diego, entitled "PMS, the Menopause and You." Their enthusiasm and endorsement of this work is a regular source of inspiration.

We owe a huge debt to our wives, who have put up with our constant preoccupation with this project: to Marcela for her business knowledge, her insight, her help with the book title, and for discovering our publisher, and to Aleida for her curbside legal consults.

Finally, to George Trim of North Star Publications for his teaching, his knowledge, and most of all, his honesty. We share your pride in this, the final result. May the next book be a little easier on you.

INDEX

abdominal hysterectomy, 213–14
ablation. *See* endometrial ablation
abscess, 75
abstinence, 84, 89–90, 102–103
Acquired Immunodeficiency
 Syndrome. *See* AIDS
acyclovir, 81–84
adhesions, 188, 190, 207
age concerns, 238–39
AIDS, 68, 89, 93–104
 yeast infections, 52, 54, 98–99
AIDS-Related Complex, 97
alcohol use
 breast lumps, 148
 metronidazole, 58
 osteoporosis, 120–21, 127
 pregnancy, 228, 233–34
 premenstrual syndrome, 113
 tubal pregnancy, 198
alternatives to surgery
 cancer, 208
 cervical dysplasia, 209
 D & C, 177–78
 endometrial hyperplasia,
  208–209
 endometriosis, 208
 fibroids, 203–208
 hysterectomy, 203–209
 hysteroscopy, 176–78
 menopause, 209
 oral contraceptives, 209
 ovarian cysts, 185–86
 pain, 209
 tubal pregnancy, 196–98
alternative treatments, 229

AIDS, 100–101
 menopause, 107, 128
Alzheimer's disease, 122
American Cancer Society, 143
American College of Obstetrics
 and Gynecology, 29
American Foundation for AIDS
 Research, 96
aminopterin, 235
amniocentesis, 238
amniotic fluid, 8
anatomy. *See* reproductive anatomy
anemia
 fibroids, 165
 Gn RH agonists, 168
 pregnancy, 230
 tubal pregnancies, 193
anesthesia, 179
angiotensin-converting enzyme
 inhibitors, 235
antibiotics, 235
 AIDS, 100–101
 bacterial vaginosis, 57–59
 bladder infections, 139–41
 chlamydia, 72
 gonorrhea, 73–74
 herpes, 82
 hormonal methods of contraception, 26
 surgery, 178
 syphilis, 87
 yeast infections, 52, 54
antidepressants, 43, 114–15, 235
antiviral drugs, 99–100

oral contraceptives, 29
pregnancy, 228, 231–33
yeast infections, 52, 55
diagnosis
AIDS, 97–98
bacterial vaginosis, 57
bladder infections, 139
breast lumps, 144–46
chlamydia, 71–72
condyloma, 77
dysfunctional uterine bleeding,
181–82
endometriosis, 160
fibroids, 165–66
gonorrhea, 72–74
herpes, 81
HIV, 97–98
premenstrual syndrome, 112
syphilis, 86
trichomoniasis, 60
tubal pregnancies, 193–95
vaginitis, 62
yeast infections, 53
diaphragms, 23–24, 63, 141
diet
bladder infections, 141
breast cancer, 143
breast lumps, 146, 148
hot flashes, 128
menopause, 121, 128
pregnancy, 227–28
premenstrual syndrome, 113,
115
surgery, 220
discharge. *See* vaginal discharge
diuretics, 114
Doc Talk, xii
doctor visits, 156, 164, 169, 221,
243–46
douching, 54, 59
drug resistance, 54–55
drug use, 102, 233–34
See also medications

dryness. *See* vaginal dryness
dysfunctional uterine bleeding,
176–78, 181–82

ectopic pregnancy. *See* tubal pregnancy
eggs, 10–11, 12fig, 110
Depo-Provera, 31
fertilization, 8
menopause, 118
ELISA, 98
encephalitis, 80
endometrial ablation, 166–67, 182,
205–206
endometriomas, 184
endometriosis, 133, 157–64, 202,
211–12
endometritis, 193
endometrium, 8, 12fig, 110
biopsy, 125, 176, 181–82
cancer, 121–22
D & C, 176–78
Depo-Provera, 31
hyperplasia, 202
menopause, 118
menstrual cycle, 11
Morning-After Pill, 30
Norplant, 32–33
oral contraceptives, 29
ThermaChoice, 207
Enzyme Immuno-Assay (EIA), 71
Enzyme-Linked Immunosorbent
Assay, 98
Erlich, Paul, 87
estrogen, 1, 12, 123–24, 168
bladder infections, 137
breast lumps, 146
cancer, 121–22
fibroids, 165
Gn RH agonists, 162, 167–68
heart disease, 118–19
hysterectomy, 212, 218

New Releases from North Star

The Shadow Side of Intimate Relationships
What's Going on Behind the Scenes
Douglas and Naomi Moseley

"Doug and Naomi Moseley are experts when it comes to the underbelly (shadow side) of relationships. This book is a must read for folks who desire a deeper understanding of marriage dynamics."
—John Bradshaw

"A real book for real people who are lost in a power struggle and want to find their way to love and passion in marriage."
—John Gray, Ph.D.
Author, *Men Are from Mars,*
Women Are from Venus

"Douglas and Naomi Moseley share their amazing wisdom . . . that can be utilized to transform a ho-hum marriage into a magnificent one."
—Krysta Kavenaugh
Managing Editor, *Marriage* Magazine

Dear Cara: Letters from Otto Frank
Anne's Father Shares His Wisdom
Cara Weiss Wilson

Otto Frank motivated people around the world to carry on Anne's message of love and hope. This remarkable story can renew your faith in the possibility of forgiveness.

"You will love Dear Cara: Letters from Otto Frank! It's a story of anguish, love, nurturing, loss and wisdom—all in one immensely readable book."
—B. Probstein
Author, *Healing Now*
and *Return to Center*

Coming in 2001 from North Star

If I Should Die Before I Wake
Death: A Certainty to Ponder
Margo Drummond

The meaning of our personal death is something each of us wants and needs to penetrate. Drummond presents solid facts and wide-ranging perspectives regarding the choices we encounter as we consider the consequences of personal death which hampers our ability to pursue the best uses of our talents and of our time.

––––––––––––––

"This book 'humanizes' dying and will be an important source of information for individuals interested in the topic either from an academic or a personal point of view."

—E. Darracott Vaughan, Jr., M.D.
New York Presbyterian Hospital